YOGA EXERCISES
FOR BEGINNERS

YOGA
FLOW!

50 Yoga Flow Exercises For Flexibility and Strength

Tianna Snow

Table of Contents

PART I

Restorative Yoga Exercise #1

30 Minutes – 5 Poses

How to Set Up

You will need:

- 2 blocks/bricks
- 1 bolster
- 2 blankets
- 1 eye pillow
- 1 yoga mat
- 1 chair

Find a quiet and peaceful place to practice. Practicing in a dark or room with low light is best. Place your mat in an open and spacious area. Grab each prop and lay them next to your mat within arm's reach.

Pose #1 - Meditation

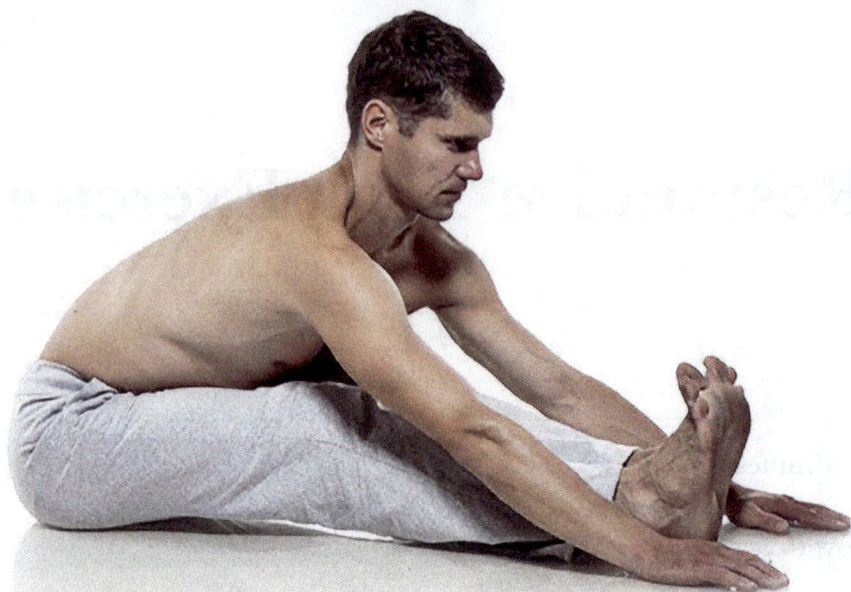

Begin in any comfortable seated position with one of the short edges of your mat against a wall. By placing your mat up against the wall at the beginning of each yoga practice, you will minimize having to move the mat multiple times.

Find your most comfortable position. You can sit on the floor, on a blanket, on your mat, in a chair, on a bolster, on a block, etc. Just make sure that you are in some form of a seated position. You're welcome to cross your legs, extend them straight in front of you, etc. Whatever feels the most comfortable and can help you to create a calm and relaxing space around your body.

(Refer to the "Hands to Heart" pose detailed in Chapter 1 "Yoga Poses.")

Meditation is a time to soften your body and bring awareness to your mind. Your meditation should be created specifically for you and no one else. It is your time to give your thoughts some much needed attention.

Close your eyes, begin to feel your breath. Touch your hands to your stomach to generate a deeper feel. Notice how your breath moves your body. Feel your body begin to create its own rhythm, flow and pace as you breath in through your nose and out through your mouth.

Take a few minutes to continue exhaling and inhaling, letting your heart rate settle into a solid pace. Feel free to quietly repeat a sound or to hum after each breath. Anything that provides a pace for you to follow as your continue to breath. These sounds are called "mantras" and can be quietly vocalized throughout your yoga session. If you are following the direction of an instructor, listen to their cues to release your mantra sounds.

Meditation can last as long as you would like it to last. If you have a specific amount of time allotted for your yoga routine (this routine is 30 minutes), try to give yourself about five minutes to sink into a state of meditation before beginning the following poses.

Pose #2 – Reclined with Bent Knees

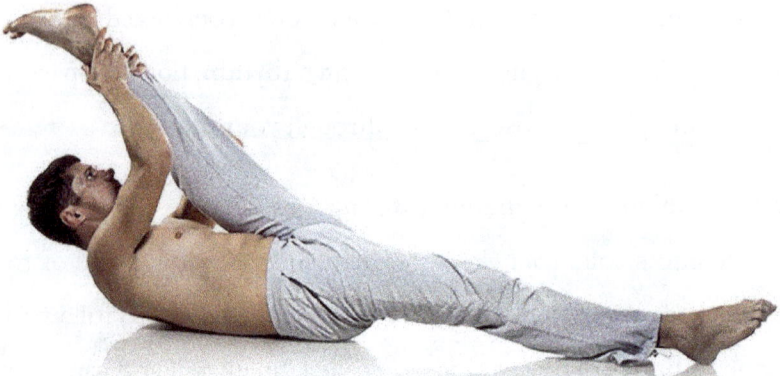

Use two blocks to support your bolster from moving backward. Or, if possible, place the shorter edge of your yoga mat up against an empty wall. Place the wide edge of the bolster up against that wall.

Begin in a seated position with your back facing the lower edge of your bolster. Place your lower back close enough to touch the bolster and bend your legs.

Slowly roll your lower body down onto the base of the inclined bolster. Inhale and exhale. Tuck your torso and fold your chin to your chest. These subtle movements will help to elongate your spine while rolling into the position on your incline. Gently roll your back down one vertebrae at a time onto the incline. Under each bent knee place a rolled blanket to support the knee.

Bring the soles of your feet together

Stack your blankets on each side to rest your elbows. Once you are comfortable, place a blanket over your body. Lean back onto the bolster using a blanket to support your head.

Place an eye pillow or scarf over your eyes and forehead to darken the space around you. Go ahead and rest your hands on your stomach. You can lace your fingers together or simply just place one hand on top of the other. Begin to feel you breath move your stomach up and down.

Restorative poses can last as long as you would like them to last. You are welcome to set a timer or simply just rest until you feel it is time to move on.

Pose #3 – Reclined with Legs Straight

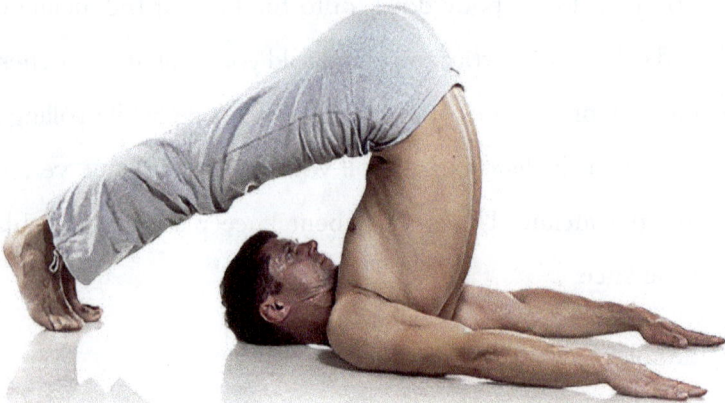

This pose begins very much like Pose #2. However, in this pose you will straighten your legs and prop either your block or your folded blanket under your knees or your legs. Your heels may feel pressure in this pose. Feel free to fold another blanket and prop it under the heels of both feet. If desired, cover yourself with your blanket and place your eye pillow or scarf in the same position, over your eyes and forehead. Sink into the restorative pose for as long as needed.

Pose #4 – Reclined with Legs on Chair

Props will change with this pose. Begin by removing everything from your mat. Let's start with a clean slate. Place your chair at the short end of your mat. Place two of the chair's legs on the mat to avoid slipping during this pose. If you have enough space, go ahead and put all four legs on the mat for optimal safety.

Place a folded blanket next to the chair as you lay down in supine position, on your back. The blanket should be long enough so that your shoulders are still on the mat when laying down. Make sure the blanket is wide enough for you to lay your entire body down on the mat. Drape the second blanket over the seat of the chair.

If you have extra blankets, fold them and place next to your mat, one for each elbow. Fold another blanket to use under your head as a cushion. If you do not have extra blankets, towels or small pillows will work as well.

Have two blankets close by before you put your feet up on the chair. Use one blanket to cover your feet and legs.

Begin in a seated position facing the open seat of your chair. Slowly roll down one vertebrae at a time with your back flat on your blanket. Bend your knees and place both calves flat on the seat of the chair. Grab the blankets for your elbows and head and place them accordingly. If the forehead tilts back, then place the blanket under the head and neck, but not the shoulders.

Place your eye pillow or scarf on your eyes and forehead.

Relax into the reclined chair pose.

To come out of the pose, slowly lower both legs back down to your mat. Move the chair as needed and transition to svasana, or corpse pose.

Pose #5 - Savasana

Relax in supine position on your mat. Let your arms float to the side of your hips, palms up. Extend your legs. Move the blankets under your knees if needed.

Adjust your head and neck by lifting your head and focusing down the middle of your body. Make sure you are evenly placed on the mat.

Gently lower the head and begin to let your entire body sink into the mat or blanket below. Follow the breathing methods in the meditation practice as mentioned in Pose #1.

Restorative Yoga Exercise

#2

60 Minutes – 7 Poses

How to Setup:

You will need:

- 4 blocks/bricks

- 1 strap

- 1 bolster

- 1 blanket

- 1 yoga mat

Find a quiet and peaceful place to practice. Practicing in a dark or room with low light is best. Place your mat in an open and spacious area. Grab each prop and lay them next to your mat within arm's reach.

Pose #1

Meditation

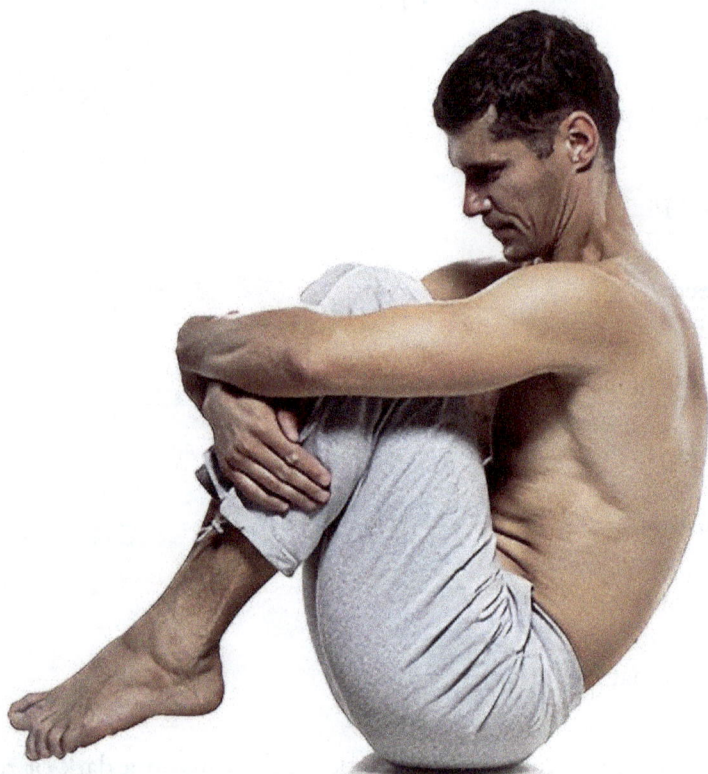

You will recognize a pattern of meditation for each Restorative exercise in this book. Beginning any yoga practice in a meditative state generates body awareness and mental focus.

To begin, place yourself in any comfortable seated position. Place one of the short edges of your mat against a wall.

Find your most comfortable position, on the floor, on a blanket, on your mat, in a chair, on a bolster, on a block, etc.

(Refer to the "Hands to Heart" pose detailed in Chapter 1 "Yoga Poses.")

Soften your body, relax each muscle and bring awareness to your mind. Listen to the sounds around your body. Can you hear other people breathing? Is the air conditioning or heat running? Are there shuffling feet outside the classroom doors? Do you hear birds or cars outside the window? Remember, this is your meditiation, your space, and your mind.

Close your eyes, begin to feel your breath. Feel your entire body move as you breath in through the nose and out through the mouth.

Pose #2

Upward Angle

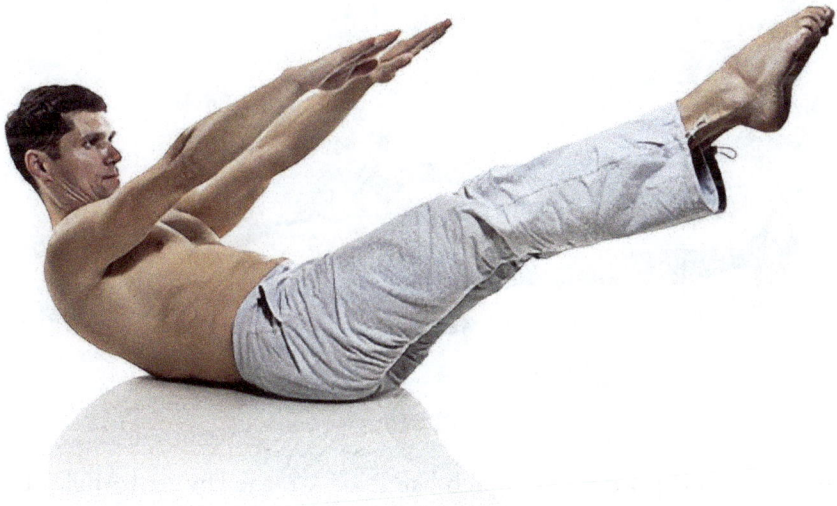

With your mat up against the empty wall, grab your strap. Make a loop in that strap. In a seated position, place your hip next to the wall.

Swing your legs up the wall and relax your torso on the floor. Place the loop in the strap around your calves. Make sure it is about midway up the calves to hold the legs.

If you have tight hamstrings (most of us do), move a few inches away from the wall. Do not strain the backs of your legs. They should be able to relax against the wall while in this pose.

Use the strap to stabilize the legs in the upward angle.

Allow your hamstrings to sink into the stretch for a few minutes. Release the straps, gently lower your legs.

Pose #3

Wide Angle

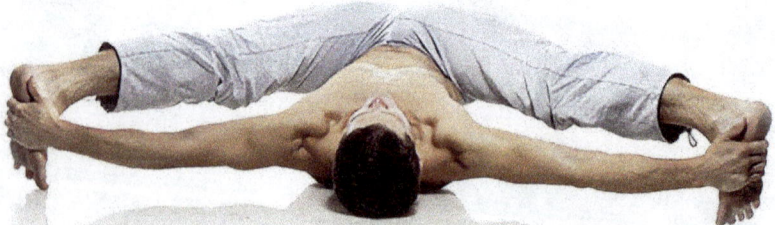

The wide angle pose is very much like Pose #2, the Upward Angle. There are a few changes.

Place two bricks on your mat and against the wall. Place your bolster against those bricks.

Sit your buttocks down on the bricks and let your lower back relax down the bolster.

Recline back on the bolster supporting your neck with your hands as needed. Roll a blanket and place it under your neck for support.

Place both of the legs straight up and flat against the wall.

Let your arms fall wide off of your mat, palms up.

Take the legs wide. Use a strap as needed. Loop the strap around one calf and hold.

Pose #4

Reclined Angle

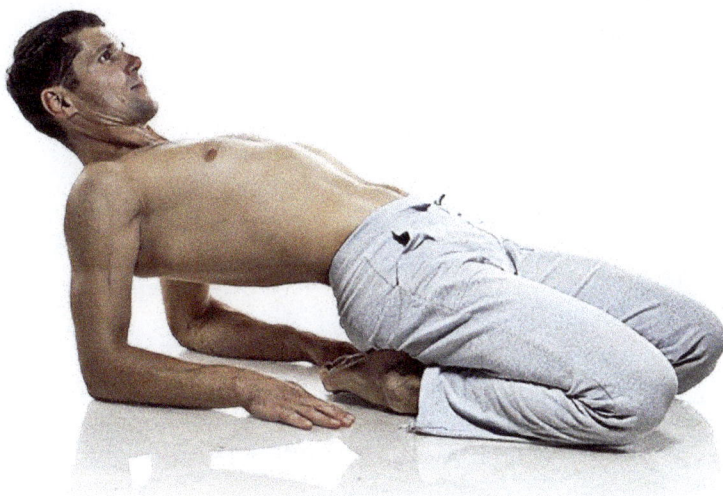

Leaving your mat in the same position, place two bricks together perpendicular to the wall. Place two more bricks within arm's reach.

Begin seated in from of the wall and place the soles of your feet evenly together. Keep your torso flat on your mat. Support your back with your bolster or with a folded blanket as needed.

Place one brick under your left hip and the last brick underneath your right hip. Gently lower both knees out to the side.

Gently allow the knees fall to the each side.

Tuck your shoulder blades and relax your neck. Lay both arms out wide. Use blanket props as needed for the neck and hands.

Stay in this pose for about five minutes.

To come out of the pose, bring your hands close to your side and close the knees. Roll to one side and press up to a seated position.

Pose #5

Front Side Body Stretch

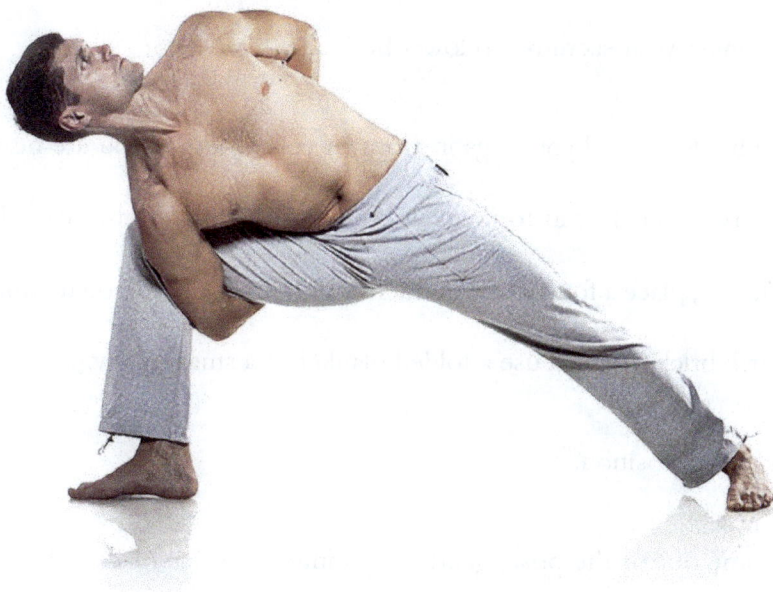

Let's grab 3-4 bricks for this one. This is an intense side stretch and will need a good amount of support for safety.

Place the bricks in a line on the center of the mat, 1 at each height, in order.

Sit in front of the first brick, then hold that brick in one hand. Bend your knees.

Begin to recline backwards over the middle brick. Continue to lay back until the shoulders reach the end of that middle brick. Allow the head to rest down onto the third brick in the row.

Put pressure on the soles of both feet. Next, place the brick that is in your hand under your sacrum and lower body area.

Continue to extend your legs in front of your body, If you are next to a wall, press your feet in to the wall keeping the heels on the floor. If you would like, place a fourth brick underneath both calves. If you do not have a fourth brick, you can use a folded blanket or a small pillow.

Rest in this position.

To come out of the pose, gently press into the soles of your feet, bend your knees and roll into a seated position.

Pose #6

Bridge Pose on Blocks

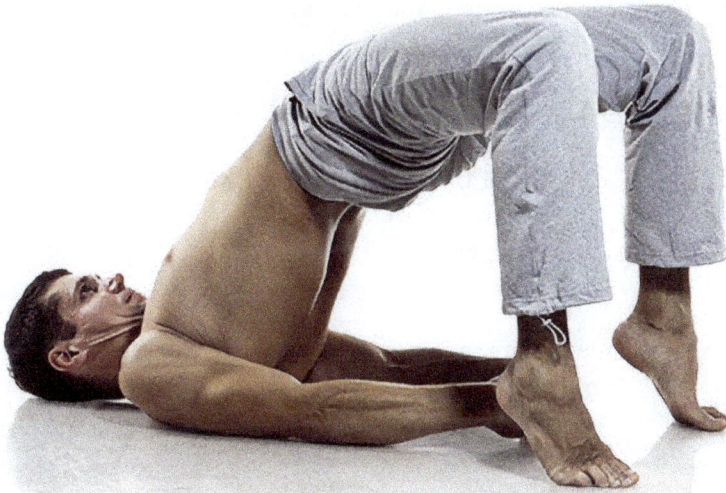

Let's grab four blocks and your blanket for this pose. Take the first two blocks and place them at a medium height in the middle of your mat. Place the third and fourths blocks at a lower height next to the first two.

Place the blanket under your lower back for sacrum support. You may want to avoid placing a blanket under your neck for this pose since you will be in an inverted position.

Next, grab the third brick and place it in your hand. Sit your buttocks in the place of the third block. Face the wall, bend your knees and place the soles of your feet flat on the floor.

Slowly lay back on the last brick. Place the bottom edge of your shoulder blades on the brick. Let the upper shoulders lay completely on the mat.

Now, you will still have that third brick in your hand. Place it under your sacrum and lower back area for optimatl support. Press through the soles of your feet and allow your upper body to rest gently on your shoulders.

Inhale and exhale while resting in this postion for a few minutes.

Pose #7 - Savasana

We will end each exercise with Savasana. It is important to transition your mind and body out of any exercise through some form of meditation or relaxation.

Let's mimic Pose #5 from Exercise #1. Feel free to modify depending on what works for you. Savasana may change for you with each routine. That is perfectly alright. Each day is different. Therefore, let your yoga practice evolve each day as well.

Relax in supine position on your mat. Let your arms float to the side of your hips, palms up. Extend your legs. Move the blankets under your knees if needed.

Adjust your head and neck by lifting your head and focusing down the middle of your body. Make sure you are evenly placed on the mat.

Gently lower the head and let your entire body sink into the mat or blanket below.

Follow the breathing methods in the meditation practice as mentioned in Part 2 of this book as well as in Pose #1 of this exercise.

Restorative Yoga

Exercise #3

75 Minutes – 6 Poses

How to Setup

You will need:

- 1 yoga mat
- 1 strap or belt
- 1 bolster

Find a quiet and peaceful place to practice. Practicing in a dark or room with low light is best. Place your mat in an open and spacious area. Grab each prop and lay them next to your mat within arm's reach.

Pose #1

Meditation

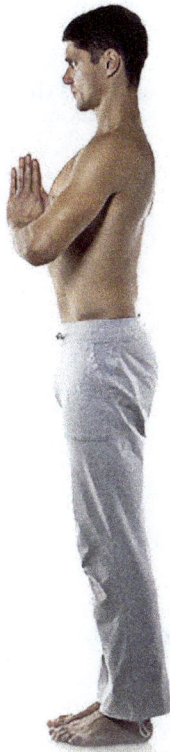

Once again, we begin in meditation. Find the most comfortable position for your body - on the floor, on a blanket, on your mat, in a chair, on a bolster, on a block, etc.

(Refer to the "Hands to Heart" pose detailed in Chapter 1 "Yoga Poses.")

Cross your legs, extend the legs, widen the legs. It's up to you. Let your hands drift softly by your side or on to the tops of your knees. You can place your hands, palms up, or palms down. As always, be comfortable.

Close your eyes, begin to feel your breath. Touch your hands to your stomach to generate a deeper feel for how your breath moves your body. Feel your body begin to create its own rhythm, flow and pace yourself as you breath in through your nose and out through your mouth.

The simple act of inhaling and exhaling brings awareness to your mind and oxygen to your muscles.

Pose #2

Captured Butterfly

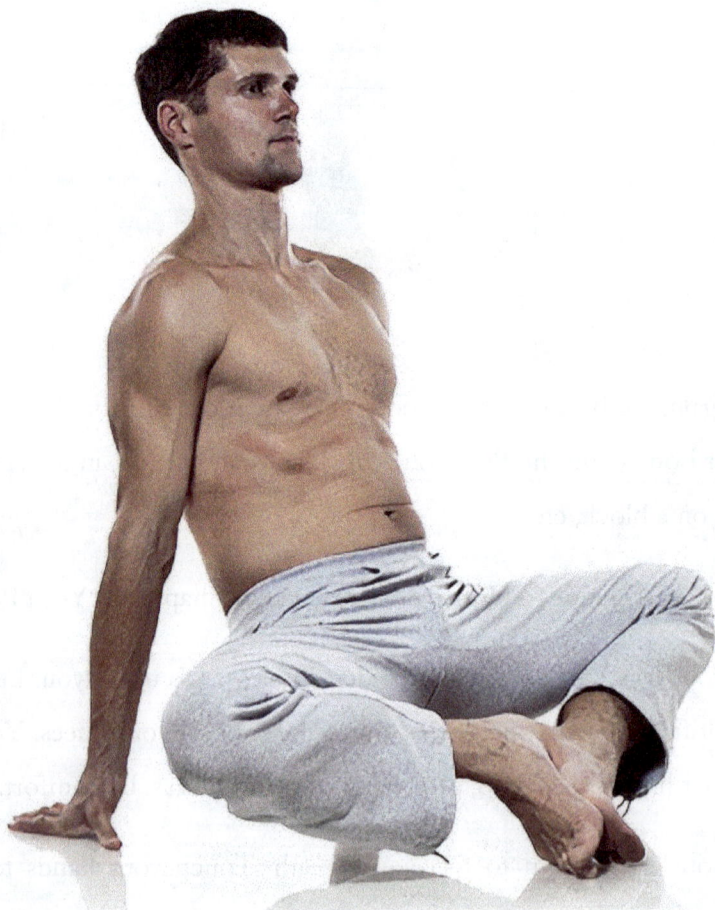

Ok, let's open up those hips! Place your bolster behind you lengthwise. Situate the bolster so that it is parallel to the long edge of your yoga mat. In a seated position, place your lower backside against that long edge of the bolster.

Grab your strap and make a wide loop at one end. Hold the tail end of your strap. Begin by placing the loop over your head and move it all the way down to your pelvic area.

Still in your seated position, bend both knees and touch the soles of both feet. Open both knees out wide, letting gravity complete the stretch. Take two of your blankets, fold them into rectangles and lay them under your knees as needed.

Swing the loop of your strap around both feet. Let it land in the middle of the sole of each foot.

Tighten your strap, and allow it to hold your legs securely in this position.

Roll down on your back onto your bolster. Remember to keep your chin pointed toward your chest and to tuck your torso as you roll down. This will lengthen your spine as you relax into the position. You can place both arms down by your side, out wide, or place them above your head. Fold a blanket and put it underneath your head or neck simply for comfort. The support will keep your neck from tilting back.

Let all of your muscles sink into this position and relax for a few minutes.

While in each position, you can return to your meditative breathing. Also, take some time to let your eyes sink back into your eye sockets to soften the face muscles.

Repeat your "ohm" sounds if desired.

Let's go ahead and come out of this pose. Gently press into your forearms to slowly lift yourself back up to a seated position.

Release the strap around your feet, lean forward and bend your knees. Slowly roll up to a seated position.

Pose #3

Mermaid

For this pose, we will need our bolster and some blankets.

Stay in your seated position, bend both knees and put both feet flat on the floor. Each foot should be about hip-distance apart.

Slowly lower both knees toward the right, and pivot your torso slightly in the same direction.

Lower the right side of your body toward the bolster. Rest on your right shoulder.

Rest your head and neck down onto your hands or your bolster below. Fold a blanket and prop your head if needed.

Close your eyes and let gravity do the rest. Let each muscle sink into your mat and your bolster. It may help to think of each muscle from your head to your toes. Begin by letting your toes loosen, then your feet, then legs, torso, chest, all the way to your forehead muscles.

After relaxing into this position, slowly press up with your hands.

Twisted positions may sometimes cause a tingling in our limbs. If this begins to happen, make sure to reposition your arms or legs to redirect the circulation.

Repeat these steps on the left side.

Pose #4

Constructive Rest Pose

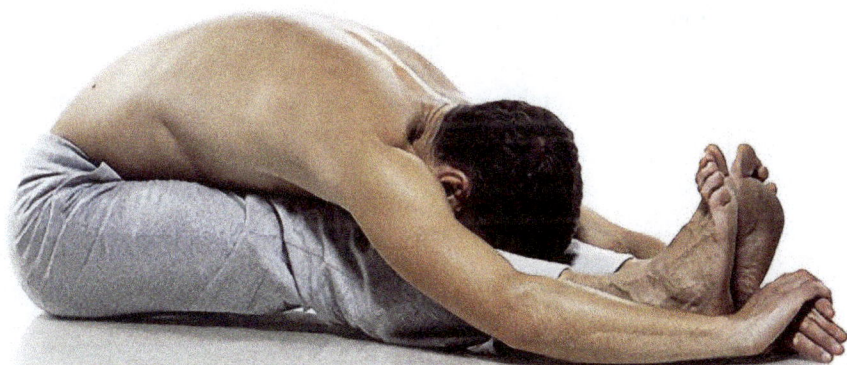

Alright, let's move our bolster out of the way for this pose. However, let's keep our strap with the loop. We will need that prop.

Grab that strap and loop it around your legs. Slide it up to your thighs, just above both knees.

Place both feet flat on the floor. Go ahead and let them rest wide, about as wide as your mat.

Tighten the strap around your legs for control. Obviously, do not tighten the strap too much. We don't want to cut off any blood circulation.

Now that your legs are in the proper position, slowly roll down, one vertebrae at a time onto your back.

Cross your right arm under your left arm, like you are giving yourself a full body hug. Relax both shoulders. This movement tends to cause us to tense our shoulders and neck areas. Lower those shoulders away from the ears.

Relax your hands and allow the wrists and forearms to hang loosely.

After a few minutes, switch arms positions.

Sink deeper into the stretch for a few more minutes. Untwist both arms and push back up to your seated position.

Pose #5

Legs Up the Wall

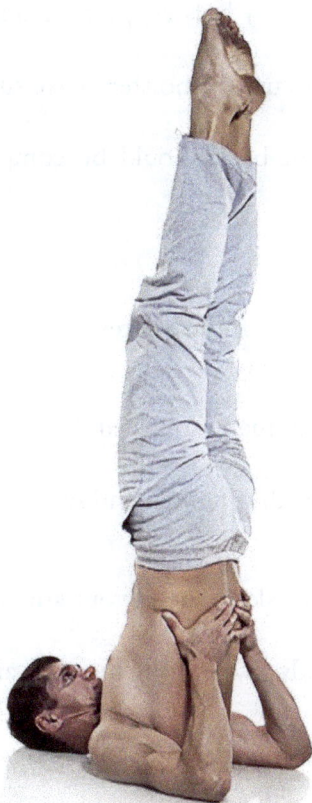

Ok, let's make our way to the wall. Make sure it's an empty wall so that nothing can fall and cause injury.

Sit facing the wall on your mat. Walk both feet up the wall. Scoot yourself closer to the wall. You can touch your lower body to the wall or slide back a few inches. Whatever is most comfortable.

Relax the knees and let your arms lay beside your hips.

If you would like to grab a bolster, place it underneath your body for support. If you decide to use the bolster, make sure that your entire upper body is horizontal. Your back should be completely supported by the bolster.

Slide your buttocks slightly off the bolster so that you are closer to the wall.

Close your eyes and continue to inhale and exhale. Feel the movement of your stomach muscles as they tighten and release.

To come out of the pose, slowly bend your kness and press your feet into the wall. Slide your body away from the wall and return to an upright position.

Pose #6 - Savasana

Now, for our favorite pose!

If needed, refer to Pose #5 from Exercise #1. Remember to modify Savasana depending on what works for you.

Relax in supine position on your mat. Let your arms float to the side of your hips, palms up. Extend your legs. Move the blankets under your knees if needed.

Adjust your head and neck by lifting your head and focusing down the middle of your body. Make sure you are evenly placed on the mat.

Gently lower the head and begin to let your entire body sink into the mat or blanket below. Soften the weight of your body and relax the muscles in your face.

Follow the breathing methods in "Meditation" as mentioned in Pose #1.

Close your eyes. Let both arms relax by your sides. Turn the palms up toward the sky. Let your body sink into this pose.

Inhale and exhale.

Enjoy this Savasana for about 5-10 minutes.

Restorative Yoga

Exercise #4

90 Minutes – 13 Poses – 3 Setup Options

How to Setup

You will need:

- 2 blocks
- 2 bolsters
- 2 blankets
- 1 yoga mat

Find a quiet and peaceful place to practice. Practicing in a dark or room with low light is best. Place your mat in an open and spacious area. Grab each prop and lay them next to your mat within arm's reach.

Situate your bolster slanting up on the edge of your mat. You are welcome to place your bolster anywhere on your mat.

Here are three exercises with different variations for props. Props may be manufactured differently. Some bolsters may be more firm than others. And, blocks and bricks may not be the exact same size. Modify poses based on how the props work with your unique physique. And, most importantly, make sure that you are comfortable.

Setup #1 With a Bolster

With a firm bolster, place a block on its side horizontally toward the edge of your mat. Lay one of the short ends of your bolster on it. This will put the highest edge of your bolster toward the edge of your mat. If you have a bolster that is softer, fold your blanket on top of the block for additional support. You can use this modification for each of the poses below.

Setup #2 – Without a Bolster

This pose can be done without a bolster. We will use a blanket for modification. So, if you don't have a bolster, fold two blankets into rectangles. Lay the blankets on top of one another. This will create a makeshift bolster. Depending on your height, add blankets as needed. It is very important to remember to modify as needed based on your body size. Place two blocks underneath the blankets if needed. This will prop each blanket up for more support. Place one block at the very back of your mat. Place a second block directly in front of the first block.

Lay each of the blankets over the blocks. The blankets will tilt upwards toward the back of the mat.

Setup #3

Place the first bolster horizontally toward the edge of your mat. Place the second bolster lengthwise along the mat. Rest the short end of that bolster on the first bolster. This will create a slanted edge and inclines the bolster.

Once you've inclined your bolster, you're ready to make yourself comfortable in the following poses.

Each of these incline setups can be used in your everyday life. You can set up on your bed while you read, on your couch while watching TV or just on the floor if you need a lower back stretch.

Pose #1 - Meditation

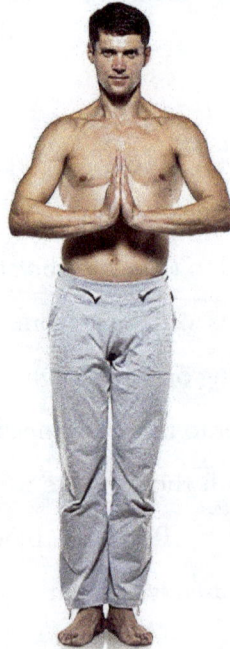

Begin in any comfortable seated position with one of the short edges of your mat against a wall. By placing your mat up against the wall at the beginning of each yoga practice, you will minimize having to move the mat multiple times.

Find your most comfortable position. You can sit on the floor, on a blanket, on your mat, in a chair, on a bolster, on a block, etc. Just make sure that you are in some form of a seated position.

(Refer to the "Hands to Heart" pose detailed in Chapter 1 "Yoga Poses.")

You are welcome to cross your legs, extend them straight out in front of you, etc. Whatever feels the most comfortable and can help you to create a calm space around your body.

Meditation is a time for you to soften your body and bring awareness to your mind. Your meditation should be created specifically for you and no one else.

Close your eyes, begin to feel your breath. Touch your hands to your stomach to generate a deeper feel for how your breath moves your body. Feel your body begin to create its own rhythm and flow as your breath in through your nose and out through your mouth.

Pose #2 - Reclining Tree Pose

In a seated position on your mat, extend your legs in front of you. Slowly roll your lower body down onto the base of the bolster. Inhale and exhale sure this motion. Tuck your torso and fold your chin to your chest. These subtle movements will help to elongate your spine while rolling into the position on your incline.

Gently roll your back one vertebrae at a time onto the incline. Support your lower body by placing your hands, palms down, on the mat beside your hips. Or, for a stronger core, straighten both arms in front of you as you lower your upper body. Rest your arms down to your mat.

After positioning yourself in an supine position on your incline, continue inhaling and exhaling. Bend your right knee. Slowly let it fall to the side of your body on your mat. Bring your right foot inward and let the sole of that foot touch your thigh. Lay both arms out to the side of your body, palms facing up. After a few minutes here, repeat on the left side.

If you need more props:

Place a blanket under your head if your neck is uncomfortable. If your chin is facing the ceiling, use the blanket for support. Fold the blanket as many times as necessary. Your neck should feel relaxed during this pose. Do not add the blanket if your neck is not strained in this position. Sometimes added support can force the neck forward, causing an awkward placement.

If your hips, thighs or any part of your lower body begin to hurt or feel pressure during this pose, place a blanket or bolster under your back or knees. The prop should alleviate any pressure in those areas. Sometimes your hands or wrists may not lay completely on the mat or floor. If this is an issue, place a blanket under both hands or wrists for more support. They should not feel strained during this pose. Your entire body should feel supported during this pose. The added support allows gravity to work and your body to sink into a completely relaxed state.

Pose #3 - Reclined Angle Pose

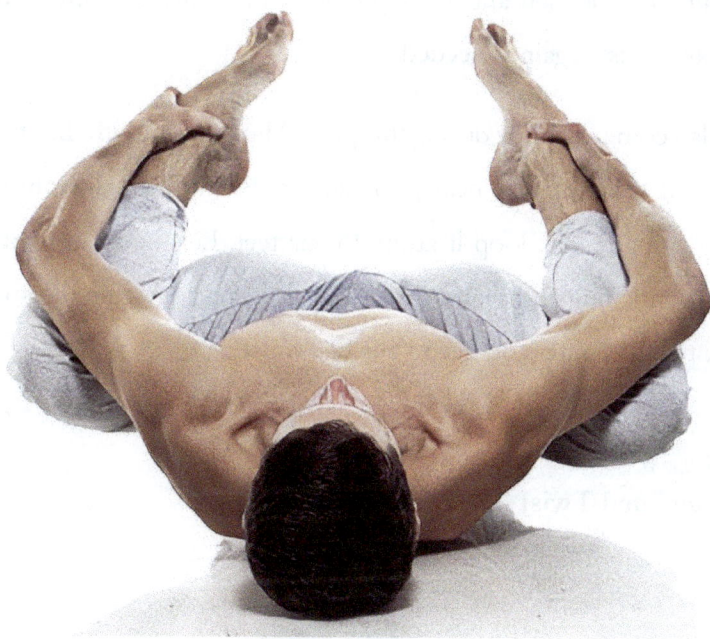

In seated position, recline down on your back onto your bolster. You will be in an inclined supine position again. Roll down slowly. Remember to tuck your torso and place your chin on your chest to elongate your spine while slowly rolling down onto your inclined bolster. Bend both of your knees and lower them onto your mat. Bring your feet together, soles touching. Your feet can be as close to your body or as far away from your body as needed. Position them so that your sacrum area feels relaxed. Lie in this position for several minutes.

If you need more props:

Once again, add a folded blanket under your head if your neck is strained. Use the blankets, bolster, or blocks under your knees or lower body. Sometimes when we position our knees outward, our inner thighs and hips will feel extra tension. Placing these support props under the tense areas allow the muscle to loosen and relax properly. Place blankets under the your hands and wrists again if needed.

Straps can also come in handy during this pose. Make a loop with the strap, slip it over your head, place it near your sacrum. Pull it through from the inside of your thighs, and loop it around your feet. Let the strap tighten slightly for a gentle hug and a supported deeper stretch. Utlizing the strap will tilt your pelvis slightly and keep your feet together.

Pose #4 - Reclined Twist

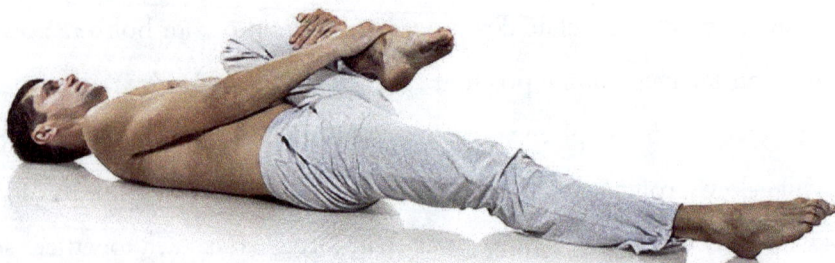

In a seated position on your mat, extend your legs in front of you. Roll your lower body down onto the base of the inclined bolster. Tuck your torso and fold your chin to your chest. Remember to continue inhaling and exhaling as your make your way down to your inclined position.

Once you are in a comfortable position on your back against your incline, bend your knees and place the soles of your feet on the mat. Make sure to keep the knees about hip-width apart. Touching both knees together, move your bent legs slowly from side to side. You don't need to touch the ground each time. Gently sway the legs left to right. After a few movements, let both legs fall to one side. Continue the same motion, and then let the knees fall to the opposite side. Repeat as desired.

If you need more props:

Add a folded blanket under your head if your neck is strained. Use the blankets, bolster, or blocks under your knees or lower body. Blankets or bolsters can be used on either side of the mat to support your knees as you drop them to the side. A blanket can also be placed in between your thighs to cushion the weight of the top leg when relaxing them to either side. Position the blanket between the knees as well if you begin to feel pressure on your joint area. Add your folded blankets for your arms, hands and wrists as needed.

Pose #5 - Supported Fish

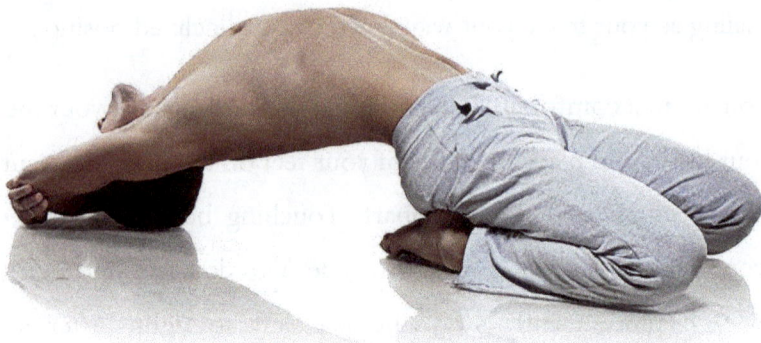

In a seated position on your mat, extend your legs in front of you. Much like the Tree pose, slowly roll your lower body down onto the base of your incline. Inhale and exhale during this motion. Tuck your torso and fold your chin to your chest. Roll back onto your incline. Extend your legs in front of your body on your mat. Relax into this position.

If you need more props:

If your neck is uncomfortable, place a blanket under your head. Roll one of your blankets and place it under your knees. This tilts and supports your lower back as you extend your legs into the stretch. Loop a strap around your ankles to keep your feet together during the pose. Place blankets under your hands, wrists and elbows as needed.

Pose #6 - Reclined Side Bend

From a reclining position on your bolster with your legs straight out in front of you, move your right foot a few inches to the right. Cross your left ankle over your right ankle. Keep your arms next to your body. You could also place your hands above or behind your head for part or all of your time in this pose.

You can also arch your upper body if your back allows the stretch. After a few minutes here, repeat on the left side.

If you need more props:

Fold a blanket or two and place it under your head for support. Blankets can also be placed under your arms and hands for proper alignment and comfort.

Pose #7 - Locust

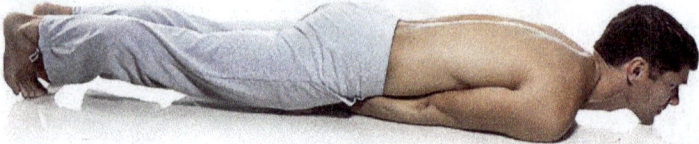

Begin in a seated position. Turn your body over and lift up on all fours – Table Top pose. Situate the bottom of your bolster next to both knees. Slowly lower your stomach to the floor. Move your shins and feet up the incline of the bolster. Stack your hands to make a pillow for your forehead. You can also fold multiple blankets as a cushion for your forehead as well.

This is a restorative back bend post. If you would like a deeper back bend, move your pelvis closer to the bolster. That way, your thighs, knees and shins will be elevated. Be very careful if you have any type of back injury. A deeper bend may not be the best option.

As you inhale and exhale, draw your stomach muscles away from the mat for a deeper stretch.

If you need more props:

You may need to place a blanket under your front hip bones for added comfort. Also, loop your strap around your ankles to hold both feet in place.

Sometimes stretching your arms behind your back releases tension in the lower back. If you would like to place your arms behind your back, place a folded blanket under your forehead. Make sure you have room to continue breathing through your nose and mouth. Place a block under the front of each shoulder for a slight lift if desired.

Pose #8 - Prone Twist

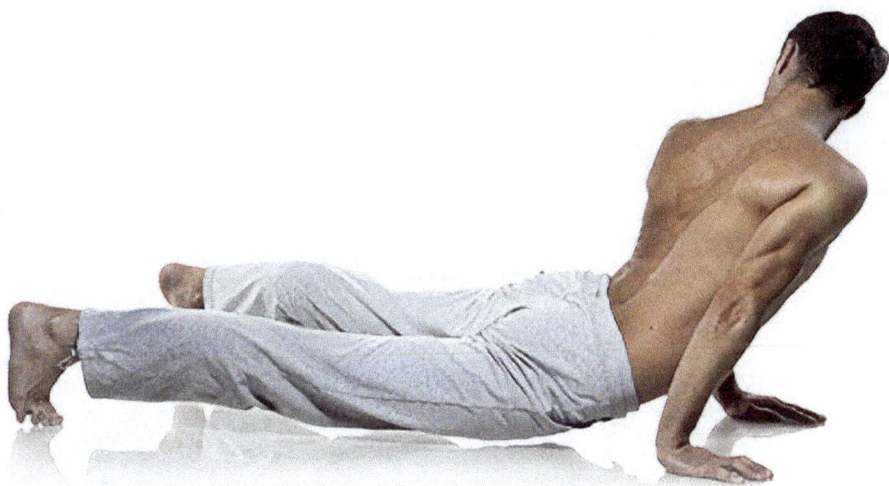

Sitting up, place your left hip against the base of the bolster. Bend both knees and point them to the left. Turn your torso toward the bolster and place both hands on the mat beside that bolster. Slowly lower your torso down. Let your chest rest softly on the incline of the bolster.

Wrap your arms around the bolster or let both arms relax beside the bolster. Lay the side of your face down onto the bolster. Either side is fine. Turn your face in the opposite direction of your knees for a deeper side stretch.

Relax into this position for a few minutes. Repeat the twist on the opposite side. If at any time you begin to feel numbness or a tingling anywhere in the body during a twist post, slowly come out of the pose. This will restore proper circulation.

If you need more props:

Fold a blanket and place it between your knees. You can also use a blanket as a cushion between your outer knee and the floor/mat.

Pose #9 - Child's Pose

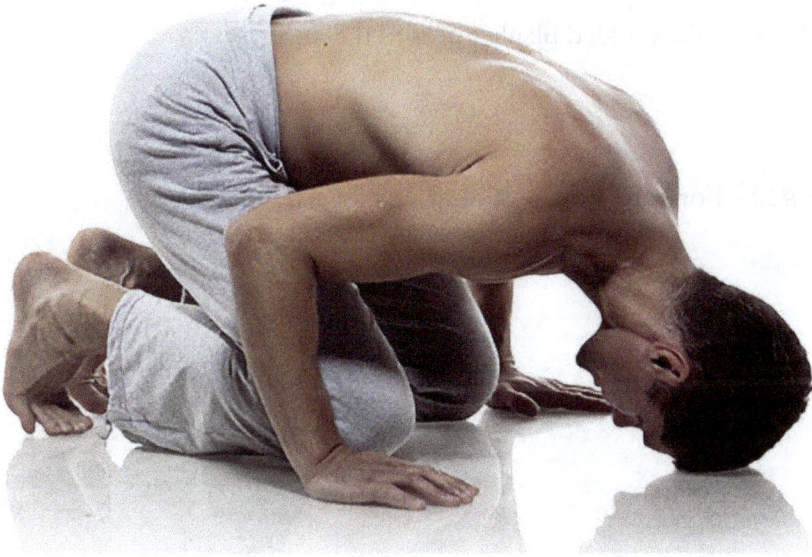

Let's stretch that lower back. Begin in table top pose – on all fours. Sit back onto your heels. Separate your knees so that you are almost straddling the lower part of the bolster. Slowly fold forward and lower your chest down to the top of the bolster. Keep your buttocks on top of your heels.

Let the shoulders relax away from your ears. Hug the bolster or slide your arms behind you, palms up.

Lay your head to one side. Relax the muscles. Lift your head and slowly turn it in the opposite direction. Continue to inhale and exhale. Feel your chest move your upper body as you breath in and out.

If you need more props:

As you lay forward, the weight of your body may create some pressure on your knees. Add a folded blanket behind the knees.

Pose #10 - Forward Fold – Wide Legs

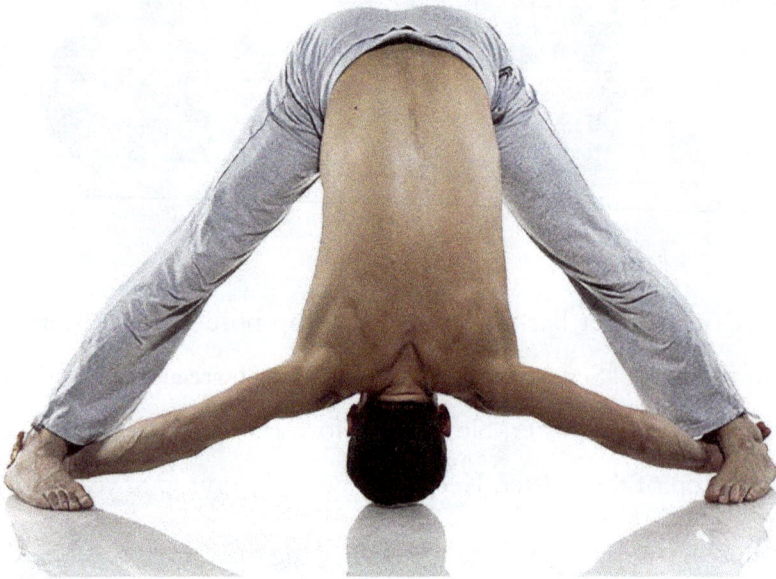

In a seated upright position, face the bolster. Widen the legs and straddle the lower part of your bolster. Your legs should be straight in this postion. Fold forward and lay your chest on top of the bolster. Stack your hands underneath your head or place a blanket as a cushion. Rest your forearms and hands on the floor. Relax your head to one side. Halfway through the pose, turn your face in the opposite direction.

If you need more props:

This forward fold may be more comfortable by adding a few folded blankets underneath your lower body. You can also fold forward in this pose with bent knees. Add a block under each knee for support if you choose this option.

Your heels may begin to feel some pressure if you have chosen to straighten both legs. If so, add folded blankets under both heels to soften the weight. Also, if your hands are uncomfortable underneath your head, use a blanket or small pillow instead.

This pose can also be done without the bolster. Sometimes the bolster can cause the hamstrings to feel strained. Move the bolster and set it up vertically. With the bolster in this position, you can rest your forehead. Set your head against the top of the bolster as you fold forward. This will relieve the tight hamstrings as well.

Pose #11 - One Leg Prop

Let's first place the bolster at the end of our mat, near our feet. Begin this pose lying down on your back. Place your head at the short edge of your mat. Move slightly to the left side of your mat. Lie down on your back with your head at the front of your mat. Place your right leg on the bolster and your left leg on the mat.

Let both arms fall to your side, palms facing up. You are also welcome to lay your hands on your stomach. Rest in this pose for a few minutes. Allow your lower back and sacrum area to sink into your mat. Remember to continue to breathe with each movement.

If you need more props:

Use a folded blanket for your neck. Support your forearms, wrists and hands with a few extra blankets as well.

Another great option: place two blocks on either side of your head. These will keep your head from turning. The placement of the blocks may also drown out distracting sounds.

Pose #12 - Cow Face

Begin in a supine position on your mat. Lay flat on your back and prop both legs on the bolster. Cross your right leg over your left leg and bend both knees. Bring your feet to the floor on either side of the bolster.

Once again, rest your hands on your stomach or alongside your body. Rest in this position for a few minutes. Repeat on the opposite side.

Remember to come out of these twisted positions if you ever begin to feel numbness or tingling in any part of the body to restore circulation.

If you need more props:

Your neck may feel strained in this position. Place a small pillow under your head for added support. You can also grab your bolster or a blanker and fold it lengthwise on your torso for comfort.

Pose #13 - Legs Up/Savasana

For the final pose, lie down on your back, bringing both legs onto the bolster. The legs should be reaching "up" the bolster incline.

Relax in supine position. Let your arms float to the side of your hips, palms up. You can also rest your hands on your stomach if that feels more comfortable. Extend your legs. Move the blankets under your knees if needed.

Adjust your head and neck by lifting your head and focusing down the middle of your body. Make sure you are evenly placed on the mat.

Gently lower the head and begin to let your entire body sink into the mat or blanket below.

Let your upper, middle and lower back "melt" into the mat. Drop both shoulders. Release the fingers and the toes. Loosen the muscles in your arms and legs. Relax the eyes back into your eye sockets. Bring awareness to your tongue. Allow the muscles in your tongue to release, and let your lips open slightly.

Follow a slow and repetitive breathing pattern. Feel your stomach move up and down with each breath.

Become aware of your thoughts. With your eyes closed, you may begin to see a certain color. Let your mind drift toward that color as your thoughts drift to the back of your mind.

Inhale and exhale. Lay back and let your body finally relax into the next few minutes of silence, calmness and serenity.

Rest in this position for as long as you please.

As you begin to come out of this pose, let your eyes slowly flutter open. Take a deep breath in through your nose and exhale through the mouth. Roll to one side, press up through the palms of your hands and return your body to a "Hands to Heart" seated position.

Namaste

PART II

YOGA POSES

Beginner Poses

Hands to Heart

Sukhasana

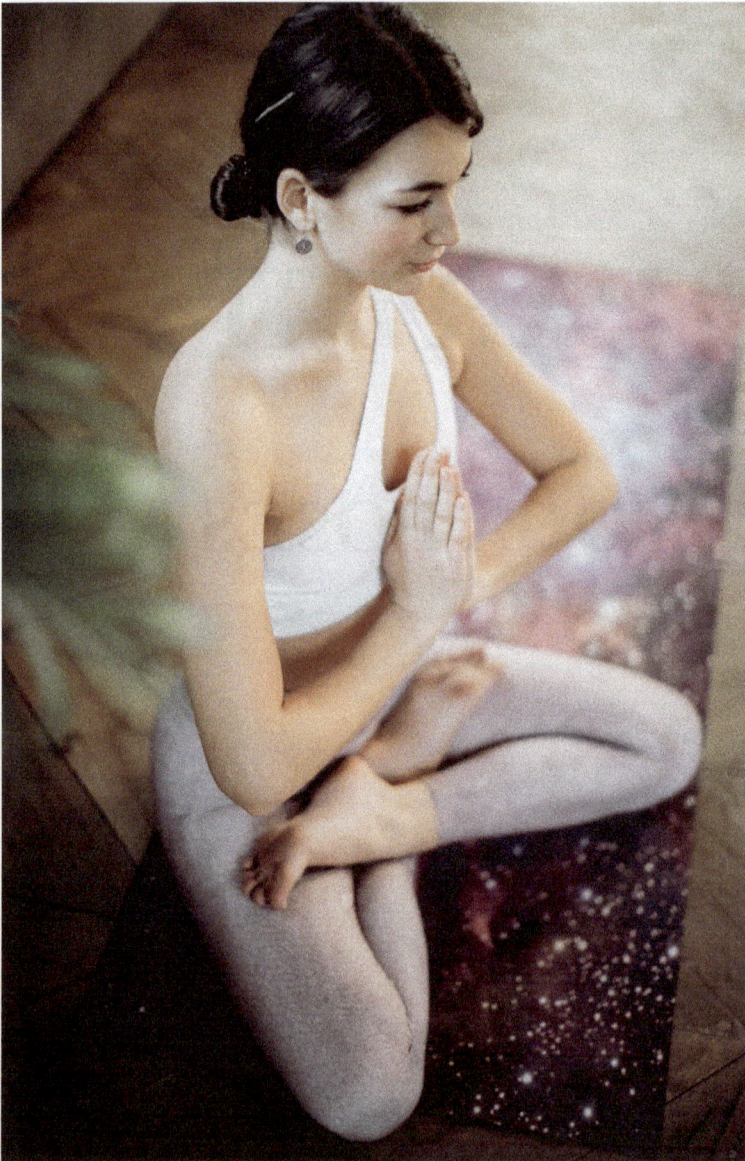

Level: Beginner

Position: Sitting

Style: Restorative, Stretch

Chakra: Root

Element: Earth Element

Anatomy Focus: Chest

In a seated position, cross your shins, widen your knees and slowly pull each foot onto the opposite thigh. Allow your knees to slowly relax towards the floor. Try not to force the movement. Let gravity do the work. Straighten your back and take a deep breath. Slowly exhale through your mouth. Place your hands together, palms touching, in front of your chest. Relax your shoulders and take another deep breath in and out through your mouth. Sukhasana can be practiced at the beginning as well as at the end of your yoga routine.

Tree

Vrksasana

Level: Beginner

Position: Standing

Style: Balance, Stretch, Strength

Chakra: Third Eye

Element: Light, Water, Earth

Anatomy Focus: Hamstrings, Hips, Knees, Quadriceps

Begin in a standing position, feet hip-width apart. Inhale and slowly bend one leg and place the bottom of the foot on the opposite inner thigh. Place your hands in Namaste, palms together in front of your chest. Exhale as you raise your hands above your head. Inhale and exhale. Gently bring your hands down to your side and lower your foot flat on the ground.

Standing   Variation

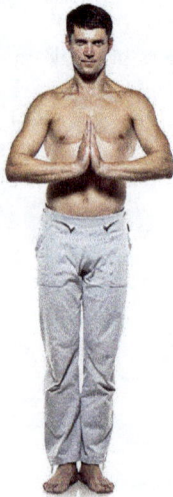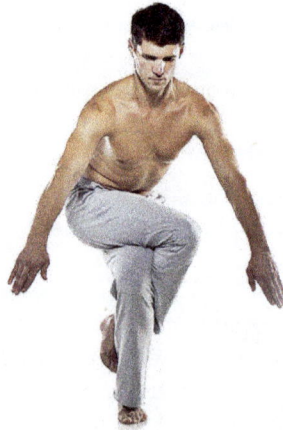

Staff

Dandasana

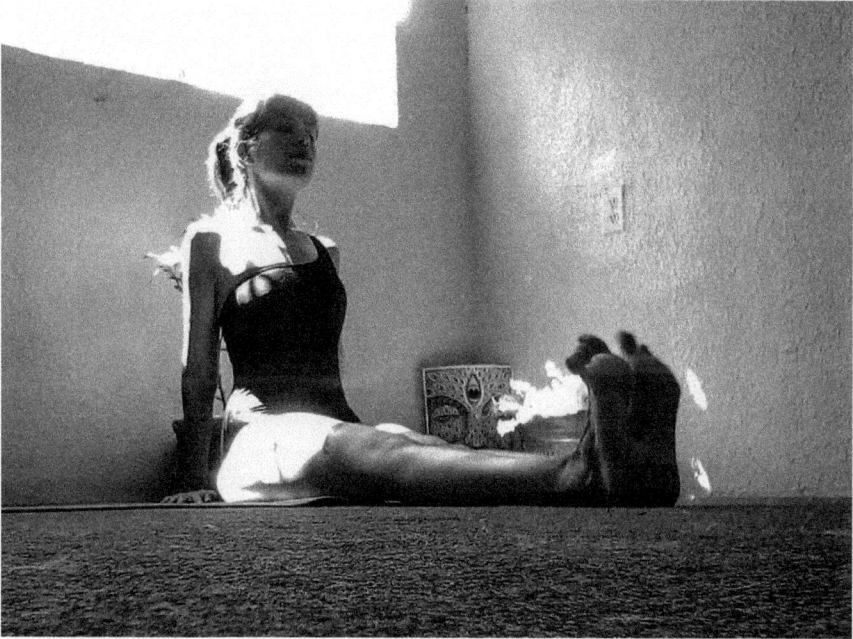

Level: Beginner

Position: Sitting

Style: Restorative, Stretch

Chakra: Solar Plexus, Sacral, Root

Element: Fire, Water, Earth

Anatomy Focus: Lower Back, Hips, Pelvis

In a seated position, inhale and exhale, straighten both legs in front of your body. Point both toes toward the sky and lower the back of both knees toward the floor. Straighten your spine, lower your shoulders and let the palms of your hands relax beside your hips. Practice breathing at a normal pace, loosening the leg muscles as you inhale and exhale.

Side Angle

Utthita Parsvakonasana

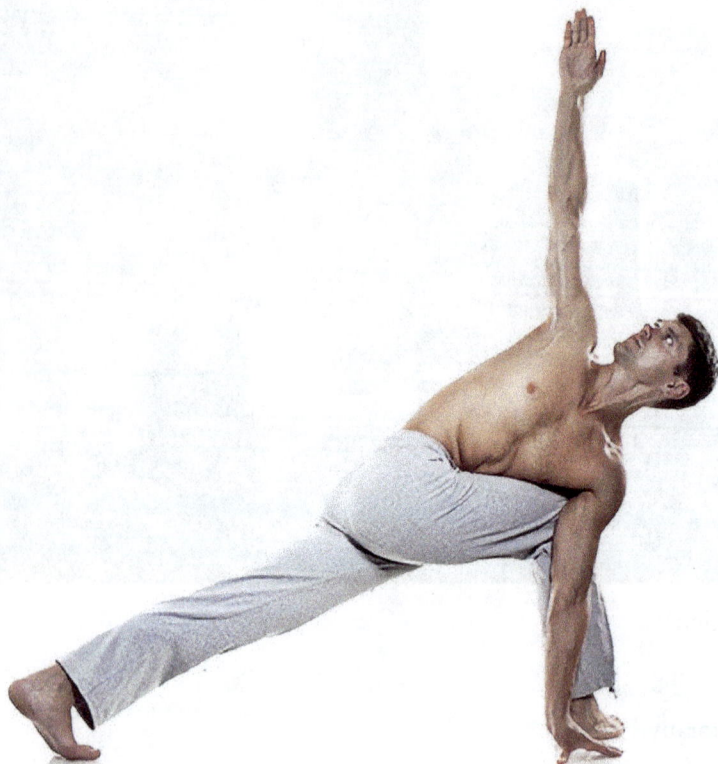

Level: Beginner

Position: Standing

Style: Side-Bend, Balance

Chakra: Heart, Sacral, Root

Element: Air, Water, Earth

Anatomy Focus: Arms and shoulders, Lower Back, Upper Back, Hamstrings, Chest, Hips, Knees, Pelvic, Psoas, Quadriceps

Begin this position in Star Pose. While rooted in Star Pose, point your right foot away from your body. Point your left foot forward, tighten your hips, engage your core and begin to bend your right knee. Inhale and exhale. Slowly shift your body to the right. As you bend, make sure that your knee is directly over your right foot. Adjust your left foot as needed to maintain balance and proper alignment. Bend your body to the right over your right knee and place your right hand firmly on the floor in front of your foot. Lift your left hand above your head and bring your gaze past your fingertips. Continue breathing normally and move back into Star pose. Keep both feet rooted firmly in the ground.

Downward Dog

Adho Mukha Svanasana

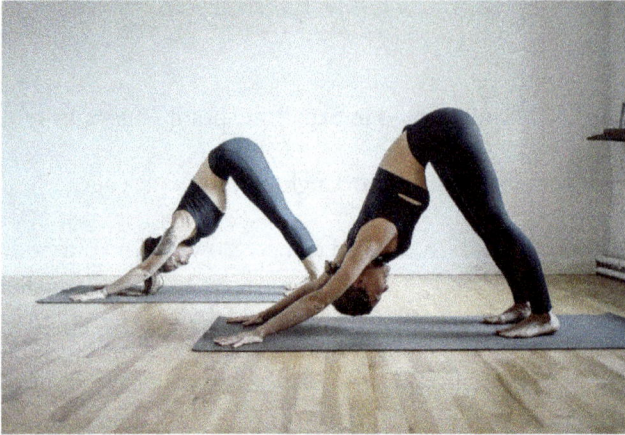

Level: Beginner

Position: Standing

Style: Inversion, Forward-Bend, Stretch, Strength

Chakra: Third Eye, Throat, Heart, Solar Plexus

Element: Light, Ether, Air, Fire

Anatomy Focus: Arms and Shoulders, Lower, Middle and Upper Back, Biceps and Triceps, Core, Feet and Ankles, Hamstrings

Begin in a standing position and lower your hands to the ground, palms placed firmly on the mat. Walk your hands out to 45 degree angle. Inhale and exhale, engaging your core and lowering your neck and head toward the mat. Turn your gaze in between your legs as you place your chin to your chest. Tighten the stomach muscles as you continue to inhale and exhale at a steady pace. Continue pointing your lower body toward the sky as you relax into the position. Inhale and exhale walking your hands back toward your body and slowly roll up to a standing position.

Upward Facing Dog

Urdhva Mukha Svanasana

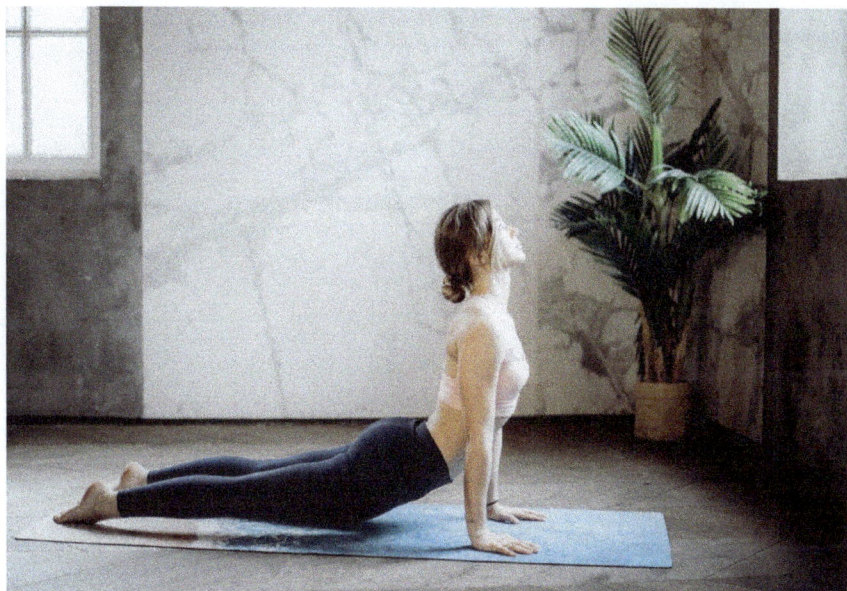

Level: Beginner

Position: Prone

Style: Back-bend, Stretch, Strength

Chakra: Throat, Heart, Solar Plexus, Sacral, Root

Element: Ether, Air, Fire, Water, Earth

Anatomy Focus: Arms and Shoulders, Lower and Middle Back, Biceps and Triceps, Core, Chest, Neck, Pelvic, Psoas

Start your pose in a prone position on your mat. Relax the stomach muscles. Inhale and exhale. Place both palms flat in front of you with your elbows bent. Press both thighs onto your mat and slowly press your hands down and lift your chest. Continue to inhale and exhale lifting until your arms and straighten your elbow. Keep both arms close to your body. Let your feet relax as you ease into the pose, breathing at a continuous pace. Slowly bend your elbows and lower your chest back down to your mat.

Thunderbolt

Vajrasana

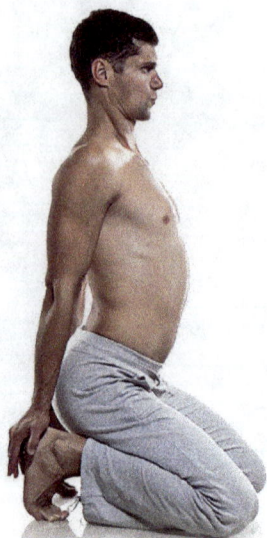

Level: Beginner

Position: Sitting

Style: Stretch

Chakra: Third Eye, Sacral, Root

Element: Light, Water, Earth

Anatomy Focus: Feet and Ankles, Knees

In a seated position, straighten both legs out in front of your body. Inhale and exhale, straightening your spine, lowering both shoulders and tightening your core muscles. Gently bend your left leg behind your body so that your foot meets your gluteus. Repeat the same movement with your right leg. Let your buttocks relax down onto both feet and place your palms on both quadriceps. Close your eyes and continue to breath at a steady pace relaxing your upper body with each inhale and exhale.

Child's

Balasana

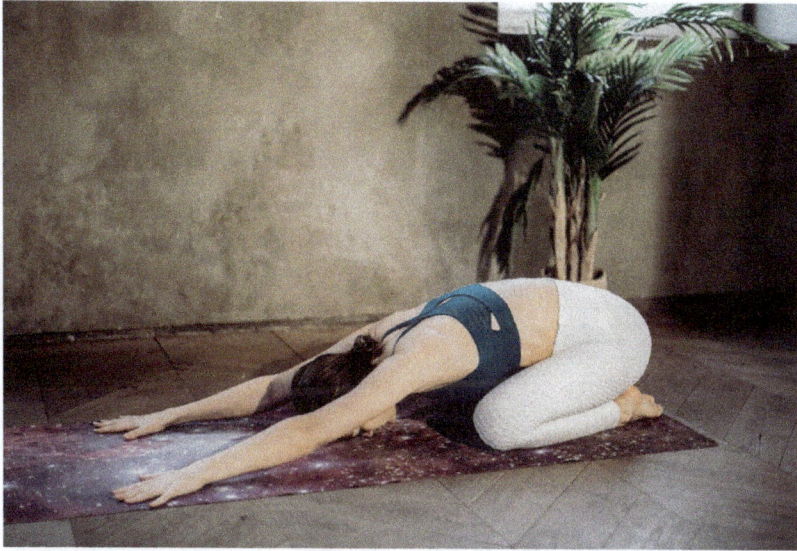

Level: Beginner

Position: Prone

Style: Restorative, Forward-Bend, Inversion

Chakra: Crown, Third Eye, Solar Plexus, Sacral, Root

Element: Thought, Light, Fire, Water, Earth

Anatomy Focus: Lower Back, Feet and Ankles, Hips, Knees, Neck

Begin by sitting in the Thunderbolt Pose. Raise your buttocks, widen your feet and lower your buttocks back down to the floor. Keep your calves and feet close to the body. Inhale and exhale folding forward and placing your forehead gently on your mat. Continue to inhale and exhale moving your arms behind you resting them next to your thighs. Palms facing up, allow both shoulders to slowly drift toward the mat. Continue breathing at a normal pace in this position and then slowly return to a seated Thunderbolt pose.

Warrior I

Virabhadrasana I

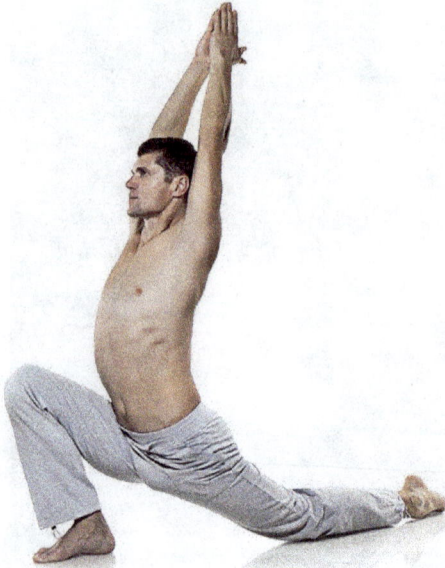

Level: Beginner

Position: Standing

Style: Stretch, Twist, Strength

Chakra: Throat, Heart, Solar Plexus, Sacral, Root

Element: Ether, Air, Fire, Water, Earth

Anatomy Focus: Lower and Middle Back, Hamstrings, Chest, Hips, Knees, Neck, Psoas, Quadriceps

Begin in Mountain Pose. Inhale and exhale and step your right foot behind your body. Place it firmly on your mat at a 20 degree angle to create the proper balance. Bend your left leg in front of your body. Make sure that your knee is placed directly above the top of your foot. Lift both arms directly above your head placing your biceps close to your ears. Continue breathing at a normal pace. Lower both shoulders and shift your gaze past your fingertips. Slowly, bring your right leg back to meet your left leg, straighten your spine and lower both arms.

Warrior II

Virabhadrasana II

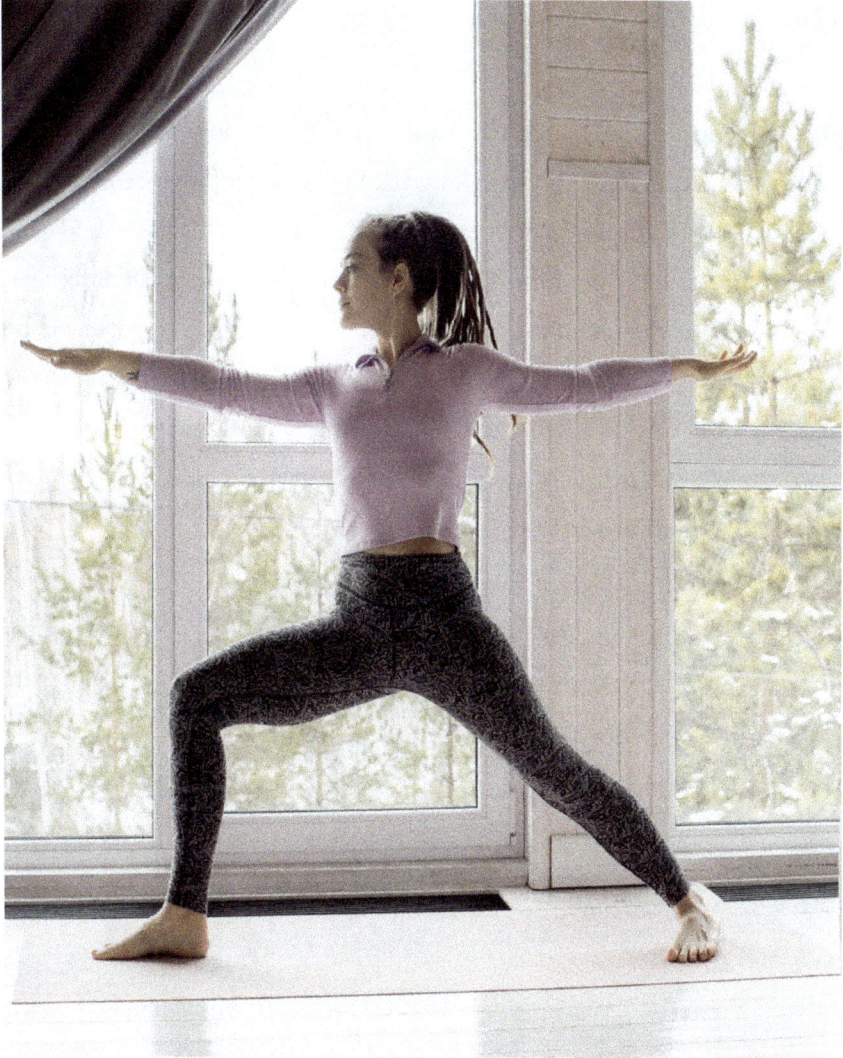

Level: Beginner

Position: Standing

Style: Stretch, Strength, Balance

Chakra: Sacral, Root

Element: Water, Earth

Anatomy Focus: Arms and Shoulders, Lower and Middle Back, Hamstrings, Chest, Hips, Knees, Psoas, Quadriceps

Begin in Mountain Pose. Inhale and exhale repositioning into Star Pose. Place both feet further than hip width apart and raise both arms to shoulder level. Point your palms down to the ground. Point your right foot away from the body and position your left foot facing forward. With your arms out wide, inhale and exhale tightening your core stomach muscles. Slowly shift your torso to the right, bending the right knee and placing it directly over the top of the foot. With a fluid movement, twist your upper body to the right and shift your gaze past your fingertips. Inhale and exhale reversing the movement to return to Star position. Gently move both feet to meet each other landing back in Mountain Pose.

Mountain

Tadasana

Level: Beginner

Position: Standing

Style: Restorative, Balance

Chakra: Sacral, Root

Element: Water, Earth

Anatomy Focus: Feet and Ankles

Standing with your feet together, straighten your spine and drop your hands to your hips. Let your shoulders relax, inhale and exhale. Engage your lower body, hips and core, pulling your navel softly toward your spine. Let your arms relax on either side of your body. Inhale through your nose and out through your mouth.

Star

Utthita Tadasana

Level: Beginner

Position: Standing

Style: Stretch

Chakra: Sacral, Root

Elements: Water, Earth

Anatomy Focus: Arms and Shoulders, Chest, Hips

Begin in Mountain Pose. Inhale and exhale widening your feet beyond hip distance. Position the soles of the feet flat on the floor. Make sure each toe is firmly placed on the ground. Lift your spine, lower both shoulders and engage your core. Tighten both legs and center the hips aligning the body for proper balance. Inhale and exhale at a normal pace and lift both arms to shoulder height. Point your fingers, palms facing downwards and lower your shoulders away from your ears. Continue breathing. Close your eyes if desired. Inhale and exhale letting your mind focus on the outward positioning while tightening your core at the same time.

Corpse

Savasana

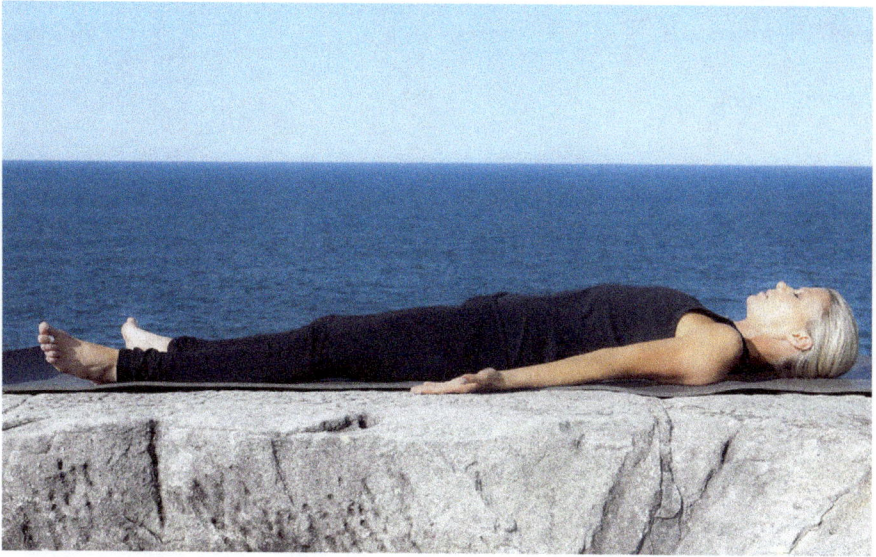

Level: Beginner

Position: Supine

Style: Restorative

Chakra: Crown, Heart

Elements: Thought, Air

Anatomy Focus: Lower Back

Begin in a seated position with both legs straight in front of your body. Lower both shoulders, tuck your lower back and place your chin to your chest. Reach both arms in front of your upper body. Inhale, exhale and slowly roll down to a supine position. Rest both arms wide beside your body with palms facing the sky. Let your feet fall the side. Allow the backs of your legs to loosen. Let your spine, neck and head melt into the mat as your breathing slows to a natural rhythm.

Butterfly

Baddha Konasana

Level: Beginner

Position: Sitting

Style: Stretch

Chakra: Sacral, Root

Element: Water, Earth

Anatomy Focus: Lower Back, Feet and Ankles, Hamstrings, Hips, Knees, Pelvic

In a seated position, lift your spine and straighent both legs in front of your body. Inhale and exhale. Bend both legs until the bottom of your feet are facing one another in front of your torso on your mat. Allow your legs to slowly relax into the seated position. Grip the each big toe with your hands. Inhale and exhale as you gently bend forward. Gaze down toward your toes. Continue inhaling and exhaling as you slowly straighten your spine back to your seated position.

Hero

Virasana

Level: Beginner

Position: Sitting

Style: Stretch

Chakra: Sacral, Root

Element: Water, Earth

Anatomy Focus: Hips, Knees, Quadriceps

Begin in Table Top position. Sit back on your buttocks resting in between both knees. Place both hands on your quadriceps, palms down. Inhale and gently lower your chin to your chest. Exhale and let your hips relax into the seated position. Continue to inhale and exhale making sure to keep your shoulders lowered and away from your ears.

Garland

Malasana

Level: Beginner

Position: Standing

Style: Stretch

Chakra: Sacral, Root

Element: Water, Earth

Anatomy Focus: Lower Back, Hamstrings, Hips, Pelvic

Begin in Mountain pose, lift your spine and engage your core. Bring your hands to Namaste, inhale and gently bend both knees lowering your buttocks to the floor. Balance on your feet and rest both elbows on your inner thighs. Inhale and exhale as you slowly place both palms on the floor to push back up to standing position. Continue breathing at a normal pace.

Cobbler

Baddha Konasana

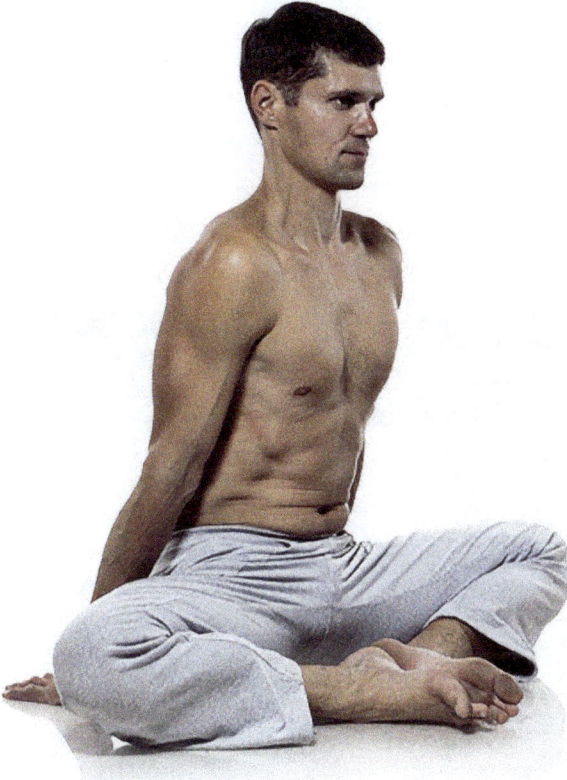

Level: Beginner

Position: Sitting

Style: Stretch

Chakra: Sacral, Root

Anatomy Focus: Lower Back, Feet and Ankles, Hamstrings, Hips, Knees, Pelvic

In a seated position, begin with your feet and legs in front of you. Inhale and exhale as you bend both knees until the bottom of your feet are touching. Allow both feet to relax on the floor and grasp each big toe firmly with your hands.

Inhale and exhale stretching both knees further toward the floor. Place both of your elbows on your thighs, bend forward gazing toward your feet. Inhale and exhale and lift your spine back to a seated position.

Chair

Utkatasana

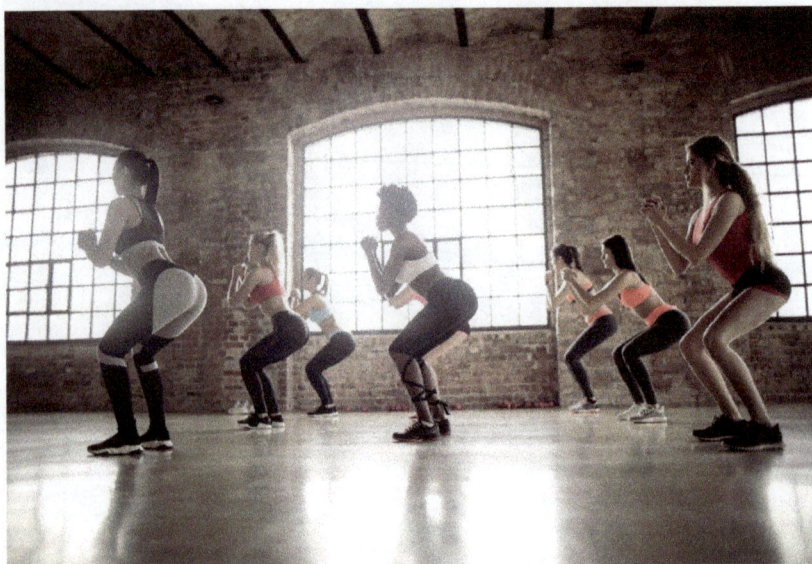

Level: Beginner

Position: Standing

Style: Forward-Bend, Stretch, Strength, Balance

Chakra: Throat, Sacral, Root

Element: Ether, Water, Earth

Anatomy Focus: Arms and Shoulders, Lower Back, Hips, Knees, Pelvic,

Quadriceps

Begin in Mountain pose. Move your feet together so that they are touching. Plant both feet firmly in the ground, focusing on the heels as well as each toe. Inhale and exhale engaging your core, lowering your shoulder and tightening the glute muscles. Bend both knees. Make sure the knees are positioned directly above the feet. Continue to inhale and exhale, lowering the buttocks slightly. Lift both arms above your head and let both biceps rest near your ears. Lower both shoulders and shift your gaze upward past your fingertips. Hold this position as you inhale and exhale. Allow the upper body to gently rest upon the lower body.

Cat

Marjaryasana

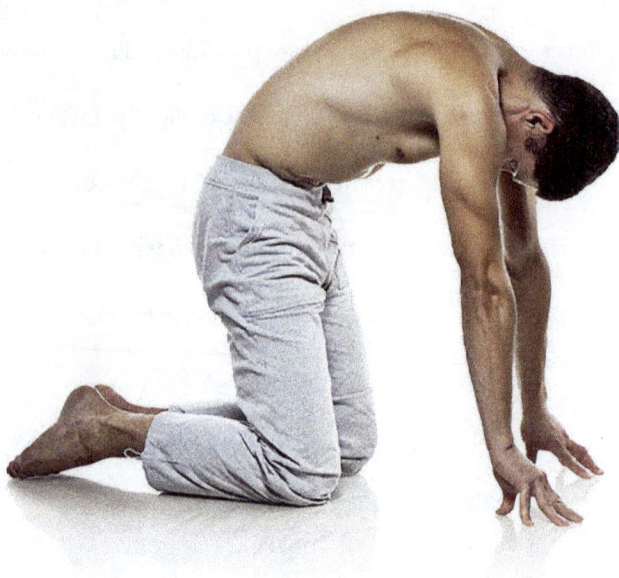

Level: Beginner

Position: Prone

Style: Forward-Bend

Chakra: Solar Plexus

Element: Fire

Anatomy Focus: Lower and Middle Back, Neck

In a seated position, move into Table Top Pose resting your body on your hands and knees. Inhale and exhale and tighten your stomach muscles. Position your feet behind you and place both palms firmly on the mat. Engage each fingertip for the proper balance and alignment. Inhale and curve your back upwards, pulling your stomach in toward the spine. Tuck your chin to your chest, relax your shoulders and exhale. Lower your back to its resting Table Top position. Continue this movement inhaling and exhaling rounding your back and loosening the back muscles.

Cow

Bitilasana

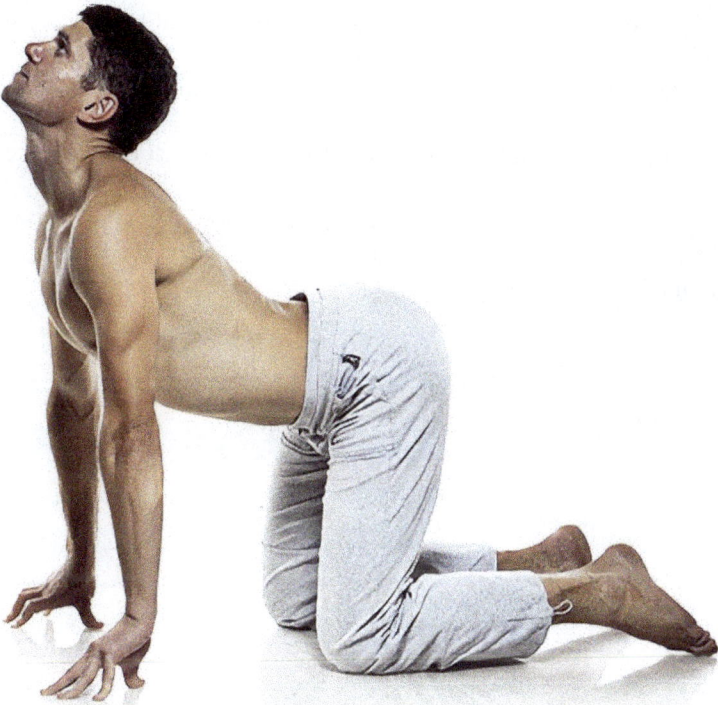

Level: Beginner

Position: Prone

Style: Back-Bend

Chakra:

Element:

Anatomy Focus: Lower Back, Knees, Neck

In a seated position, move into Table Top Pose resting your body on your hands and knees. Inhale and exhale while tightening your stomach muscles. Position your feet behind you and place both palms firmly on the mat. Engage each fingertip for the proper balance and alignment. Inhale and bring your stomach toward the floor and curving the back into a U-shape. Lift your chin and stretch your neck and face toward the sky. Lower both shoulders and exhale. Return to table Top position. Continue this movement with slow deep breaths to release tension in the lower back muscles.

Side Lunge

Skandasana

Level: Beginner

Position: Sitting

Style: Stretch, Balance

Chakra: Sacral, Root

Element: Water, Earth

Anatomy Focus: Feet and Ankles, Hamstrings, Hips, Knees, Pelvic, Quadriceps

The Side Lunge can begin in Mountain Pose or continued from the Low Lunge pose. Slowly lower your body to the floor, supporting yourself with both hands and fingertips in front you on your mat. As you lower down, bend your right leg and rest your inner thigh on the top of your right heel. Point your left leg straight out to the side of your body resting your heel on the floor, left toes pointing to the sky. Continue inhaling and exhaling engaging your stomach muscles, lowering your shoulders and tightening your glutes.

Sphinx

Niravalasana

Variation

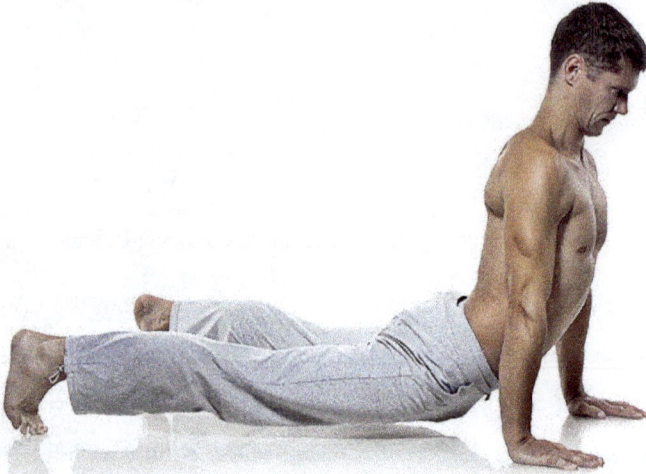

Level: Beginner

Position: Prone

Style: Back-Bend

Chakra:

Element:

Anatomy Focus: Lower Back, Biceps and Triceps, Chest

Begin in prone position. Bend both elbows keeping them close to your body, palms pushing into your mat. Keep both feet together and gently push your upper body off of your mat utilizing the triceps. Make sure to relax your neck, inhaling and exhaling during the entire stretch. Feel your stomach muscles engage toward your mat with each breath. Slowly lower back down to your met.

High Lunge

Ashta Chandrasana

Level: Beginner

Position: Standing

Style: Stretch, Strength, Balance

Chakra: Sacral, Root

Element: Water, Earth

Anatomy Focus: Arms and Shoulders, Lower and Upper Back, Hamstrings, Hips, Knees, Psoas, Quadriceps

From Downward Dog or Mountain Pose, lift both arms above your head keeping them close to your ears. Relax the shoulders. Bend your left knee and step your right foot behind your body landing on your toes. Make sure your left knee is directly above the top of the foot. And, keep your right knee slightly bent with the weight on the bottom of your right foot. Inhale and exhale continuously. Tuck your torso and engage your core on the exhale. Step your right foot forward to meet your left foot, returning to Mountain pose.

Supine Twist

Supta Matsyendrasana

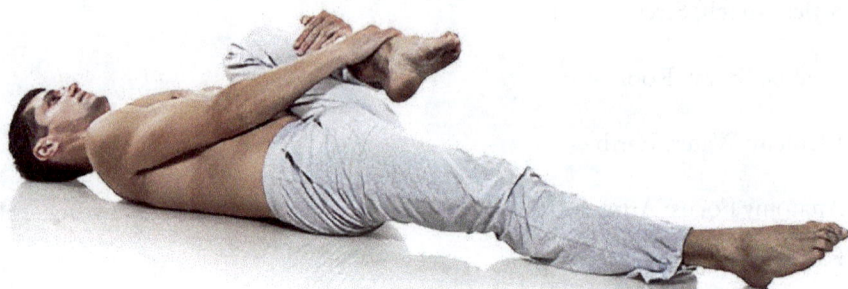

Level: Beginner

Position: Supine

Style: Twist, Stretch

Chakra: Sacral, Root

Element: Water, Earth

Anatomy Focus: Lower and Middle Back, Hamstrings, Hips, Knees, Neck

Begin by laying down flat on your back. Inhale and bend both knees into your chest. Flatten your lower back into the floor and relax both shoulders. Gently begin to drop both knees to one side of your body, relaxing one knee on top of the other. Lay both arms out wide and shift your gaze in the opposite direction. Inhale and exhale continuously through this stretch. Slowly bring both knees back to your chest and lower down to your mat.

Legs up the Wall

Viparita Karani

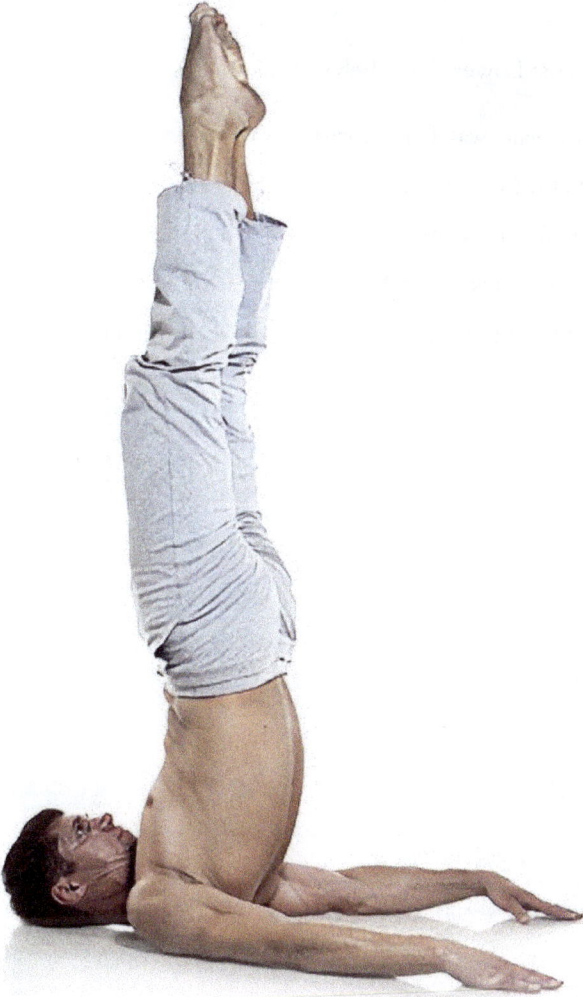

Level: Beginner

Position: Supine

Style: Restorative, Stretch

Chakra:

Element:

Anatomy Focus: Lower Back, Pelvic, Quadriceps

Find an empty wall away from mirrors or windows. Begin in supine position with both knees bent. Move your buttocks against the wall with both hands down by your side. Inhale and exhale, placing both legs flat against the wall. Relax your neck and lower back into the floor. Breath continuously through this pose allowing the blood to begin flowing in a different direction.

Sitting Forward Fold

Paschimottanasana

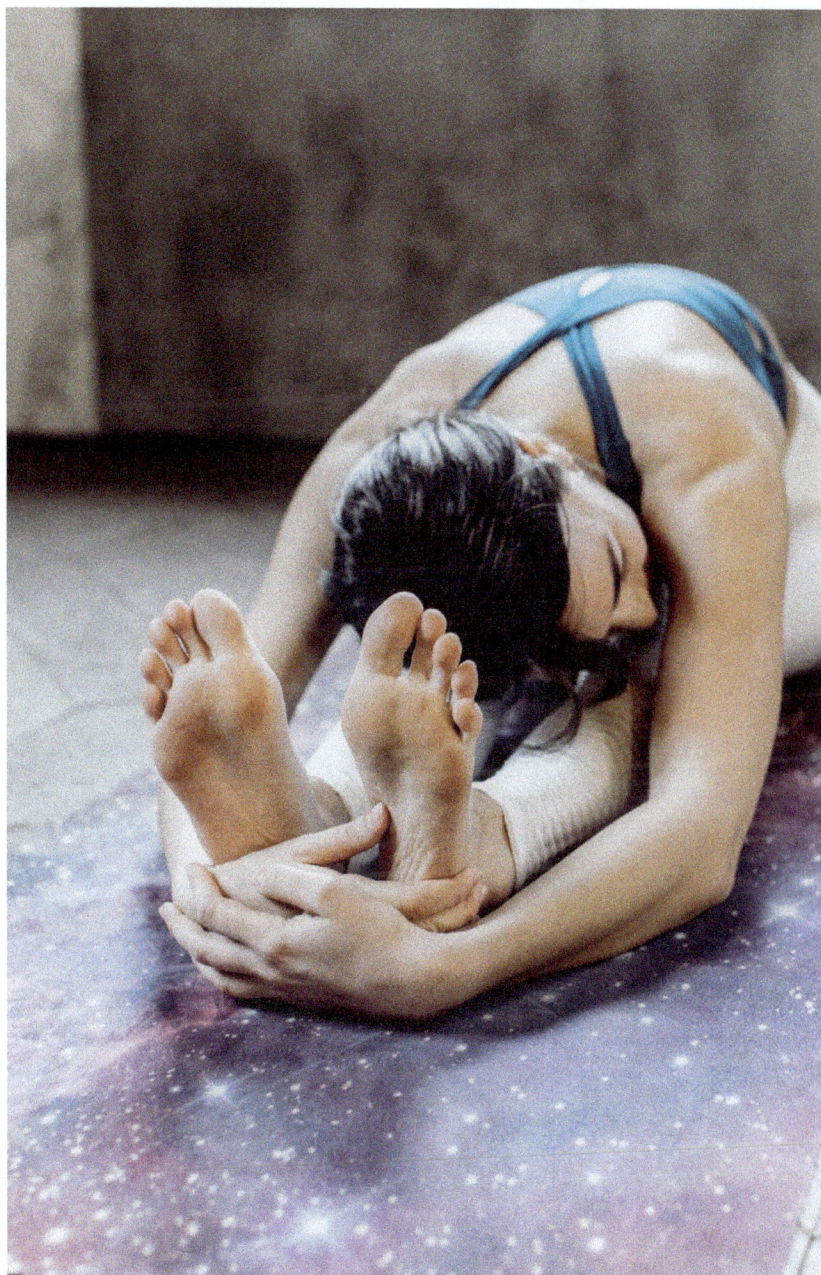

Level: Beginner

Position: Sitting

Style: Forward-Bend, Stretch

Chakra: Throat, Solar-Plexus, Root

Element: Ether, Fire, Water, Earth

Anatomy Focus: Lower and Upper Back, Hamstrings, Hips, Neck

While in Staff pose, inhale and tuck your chin to your chest. Engage your core and lower both shoulders. Beginning to create a curve at the top of your neck. Slowly roll forward one vertebrae at a time. Keeping both hands by your side for support, palms down. Roll down as far as your spine will allow without forcing the motion. Slowly roll back up returning to Staff pose.

Standing Forward Fold

Uttanasana

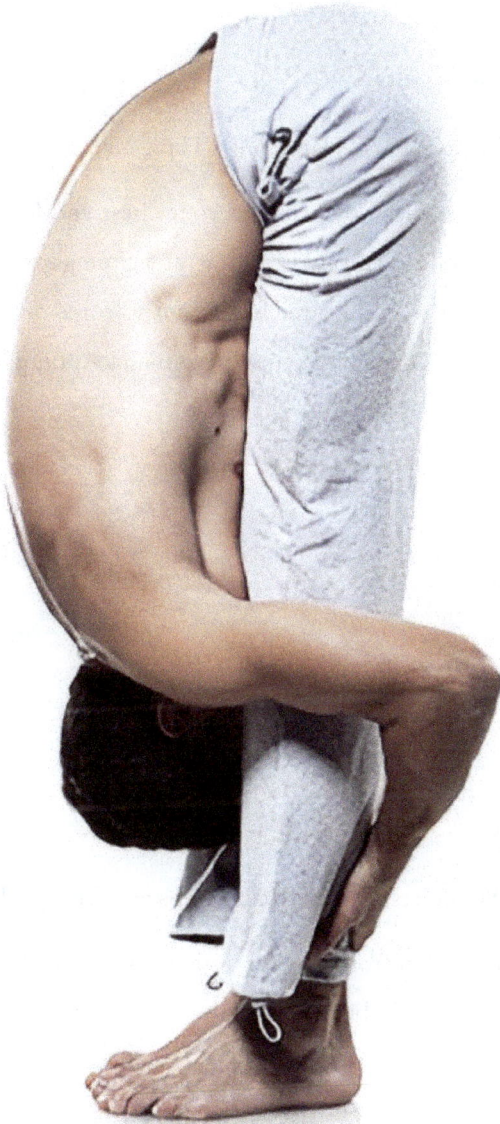

Level: Beginner

Position: Standing

Style: Forward-Bend, Stretch, Inversion

Chakra: Crown, Solar-Plexus, Sacral, Root

Element: Thought, Fire, Water, Earth

Anatomy Focus: Lower and Upper Back, Hamstrings, Hips, Neck

Begin in Mountain pose. Inhale, tuck your chin to your chest and lower both shoulders. Exhale and slowly roll down one vertebrae at a time gazing toward your toes. Allow gravity to assist with the stretch. Try not to force or push the stretch as you fold. Slowly roll back up, chin to chest, returning to Mountain pose.

Table Top

Bharmanasana

Level: Beginner

Position: Sitting

Style: Restorative

Chakra: Sacral, Root

Element: Water, Earth

Anatomy Focus: Arms and Shoulders, Lower Back, Biceps and Triceps, Knees

In Vajrasana, walk both hands out in front of your body stopping just below the shoulders. Lift up on your knees. Keep both feet on the floor. Inhale and exhale engaging your stomach muscles. Align your head and neck with your back so that your upper torso is parallel to your mat. Shift your gaze to the mat. Gently rotate back into Child's pose.

Plank

Phalakasana

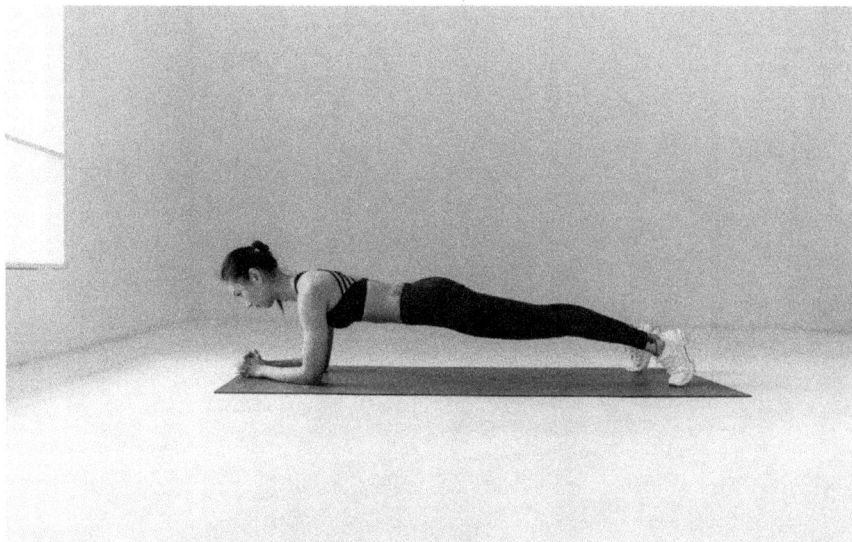

Level: Beginner

Position: Prone

Style: Strength

Chakra: Solar Plexus

Element: Fire

Anatomy Focus: Arms and Shoulders, Biceps and Triceps, Core

In Downward Dog pose, plant both feet and hands firmly on your mat, utilizing all fingertips for balance. Slowly move the entire body parallel to your mat focusing weight on the toes and hands. Make sure both hands are directly below both shoulders. Inhale and exhale through each move. Gaze toward the floor shifting the hips inward. If your wrists begin to experience a painful pressure, release to your elbows keeping your hands in front of your body. Inhale and exhale. Gently fold back to Child's pose when ready.

Bridge

Setubandha Sarvangasana

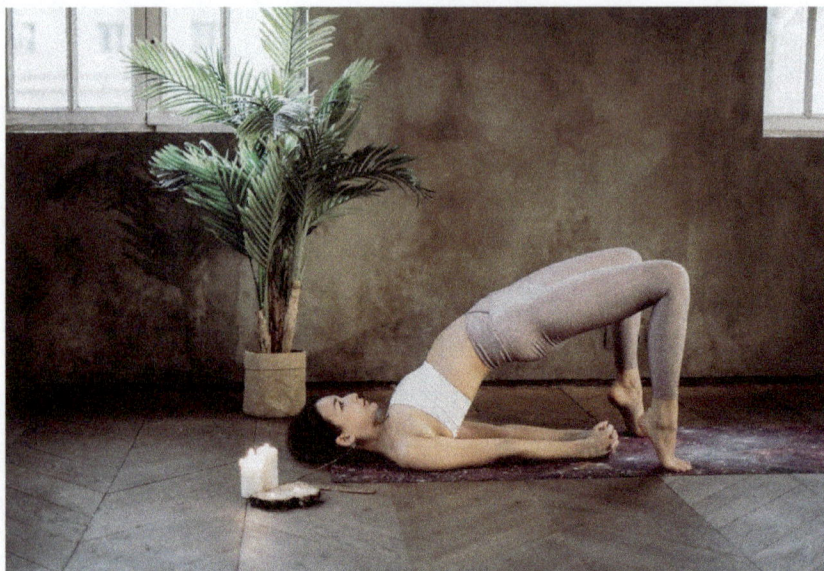

Level: Beginner

Position: Supine

Style: Back-Bend, Stretch, Strength, Balance

Chakra: Crown, Third Eye, Throat, Solar Plexus

Element: Thought, Light, Ether, Fire

Anatomy Focus: Arms and Shoulders, Lower and Upper Back, Core, Chest, Hips, Neck, Pelvic, Psoas, Quadriceps

Begin this pose in supine position. Bend both knees bringing them close to your buttocks. Place both hands by your side, palms down. Inhale and exhale, lifting the buttocks off the floor by pushing through the soles of the feet. Make sure to support your neck by keeping it flat on the mat. Lift through to your toes if desired. Slowly lower back down to your mat.

Camel

Ustrasana

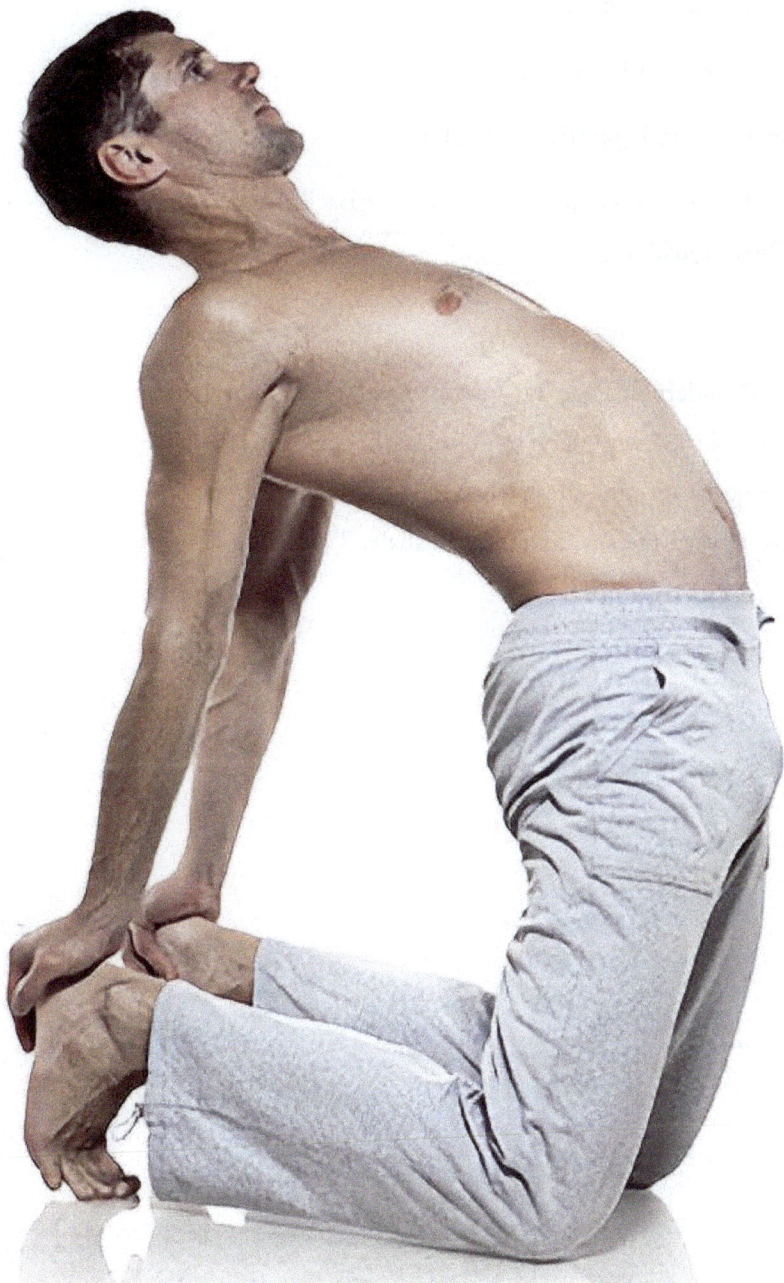

Level: Beginner

Position: Sitting

Style: Back-Bend, Stretch, Balance

Chakra: Crown, Third-Eye, Throat, Heart, Solar-Plexus

Element: Thought, Light, Ether, Air, Fire

Anatomy Focus: Lower, Middle and Upper Back, Core, Chest, Knees, Neck, Pelvic, Psoas, Quadriceps

While in Thunderbolt Pose, lift to your knees, straighten your spine and lower both shoulders. Slowly place both palms behind your body, on top of each respective heel. Open the chest, inhale, and rotate back, supporting the neck. Shift your gaze toward the sky, inhale and exhale. Tightening the quadriceps, rotate back to Thurnderbolt pose.

Four Limbed Staff Pose

Chaturanga Dandasana

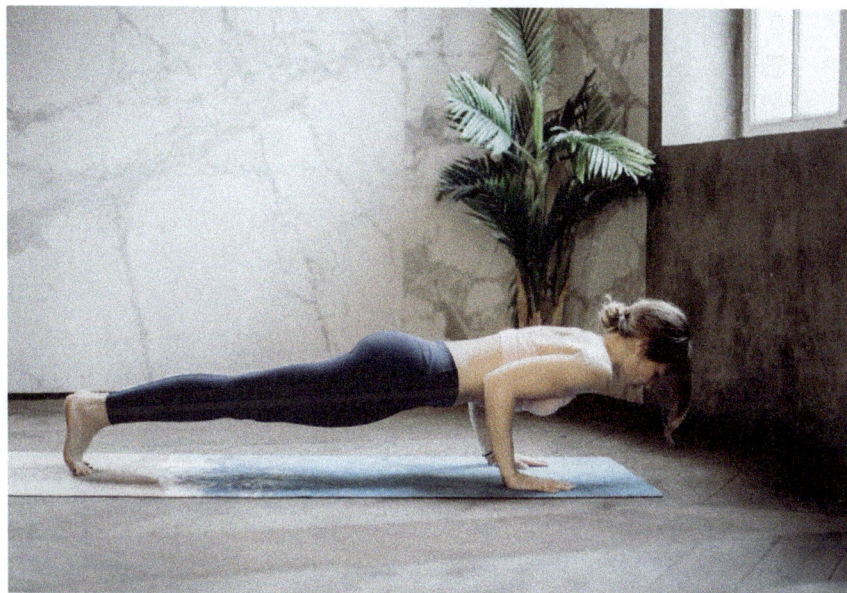

Level: Beginner

Position: Prone

Style: Strength

Chakra: Solar Plexus

Element: Fire

Anatomy Focus: Arms and Shoulders, Lowers Back, Biceps and Triceps, Core, Hamstrings, Pelvic

Begin this pose in Downward Dog and walk into Plank Pose. Find the correct balance on your toes and palms of your hands while gazing toward the floor. Take a few deep breaths, tighten your core muscles and slowly bend both elbows by your side, keeping them as close your body as possible. As you lower, keep your body parallel to the floor and exhale. Breathing continuously, push up through your palms, lower both knees and sit back into Child's Pose.

Cobra

Bhujangasana

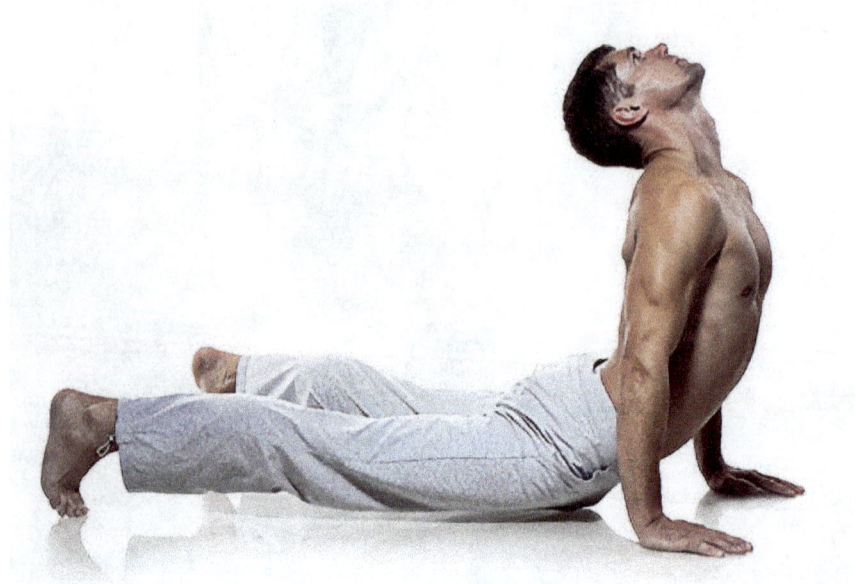

Level: Beginner

Position: Prone

Style: Back-Bend

Chakra: Throat, Heart, Solar Plexus, Sacral, Root

Element: Ether, Air, Fire, Water, Earth

Anatomy Focus: Lower, Middle and Upper Back, Biceps and Triceps, Core, Psoas

Lying on your stomach in prone position with face down, inhale and exhale tightening the stomach muscles. Firmly plant the top of your feet to the ground and place your palms close to your upper abdomen. Inhale and push through your palms, raising your chest about six inches off the ground. Exhale. Slowly lower down to your mat.

Intermediate Poses

Seated Twist

Marichyasana

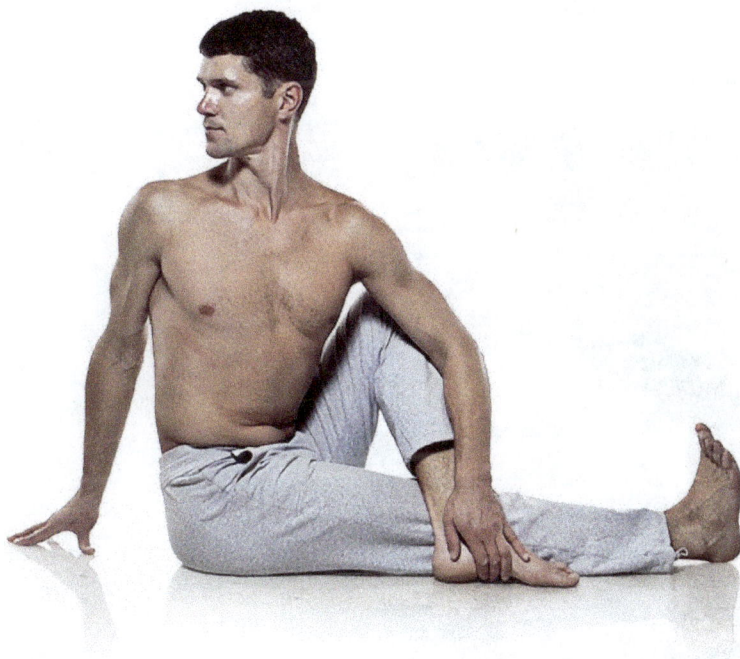

Level: Intermediate

Position: Sitting

Style: Twist, Forward-Bend, Stretch

Chakra: Solar, Sacral, Root

Element: Fire, Water, Earth

Anatomy Focus: Arms and Shoulders, Lower and Upper Back, Biceps and Triceps, Core, Hamstrings, Hips, Neck, Quadriceps

Begin in Staff Pose with feet straight out in front of your body. Inhale and exhale as your lift your right leg toward your chest. Keep your left leg straight, inhale and twist your torso as you place your left hand on the floor behind you. Bring your right arm around your right knee and slowly bend forward. Gently lift both hands behind you and lock them together. Inhale and exhale as you lower into the final position. Slowly release your hands and return to your upright seated position.

Boat

Navasana

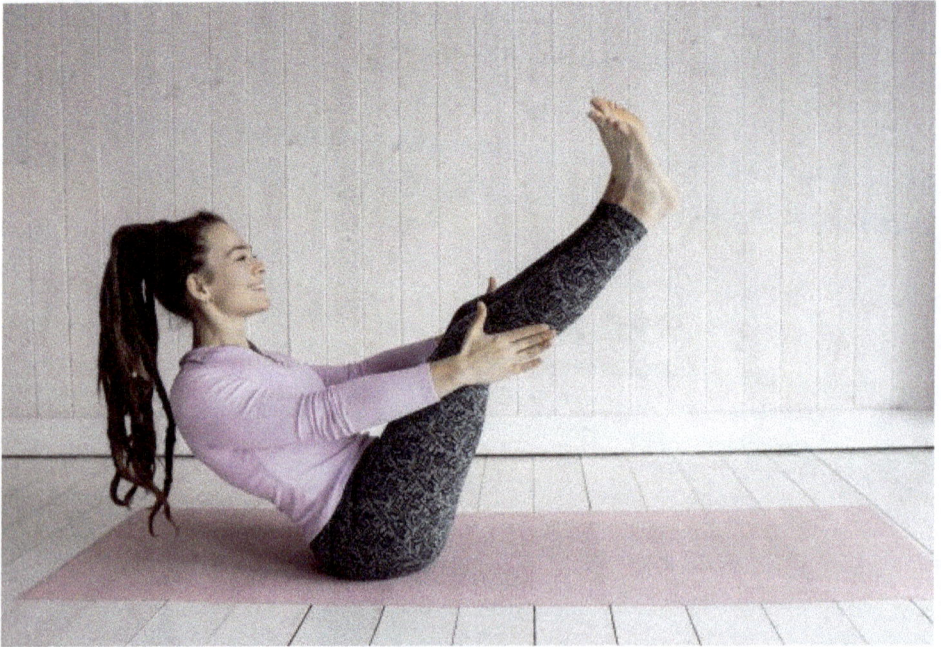

Level: Intermediate

Position: Sitting

Style: Forward Bend, Strength, Balance

Chakra: Solar Plexus

Element: Fire

Anatomy Focus: Lower Back, Core, Pelvic, Quadriceps

Begin in a seated position, inhale and exhale, pointing both legs out in front of your body. Slowly round your spine and engage your core muscles. Turn your gaze toward your knees. Inhale and exhale as you bring your legs 1-2 feet off the ground in a straight motion. Point your toes. Raise both arms and place your hands, palms facing in, to the outside of your knees. Inhale and exhale as your bring your arms and legs down slowly to the ground.

Wheel

Chakrasana

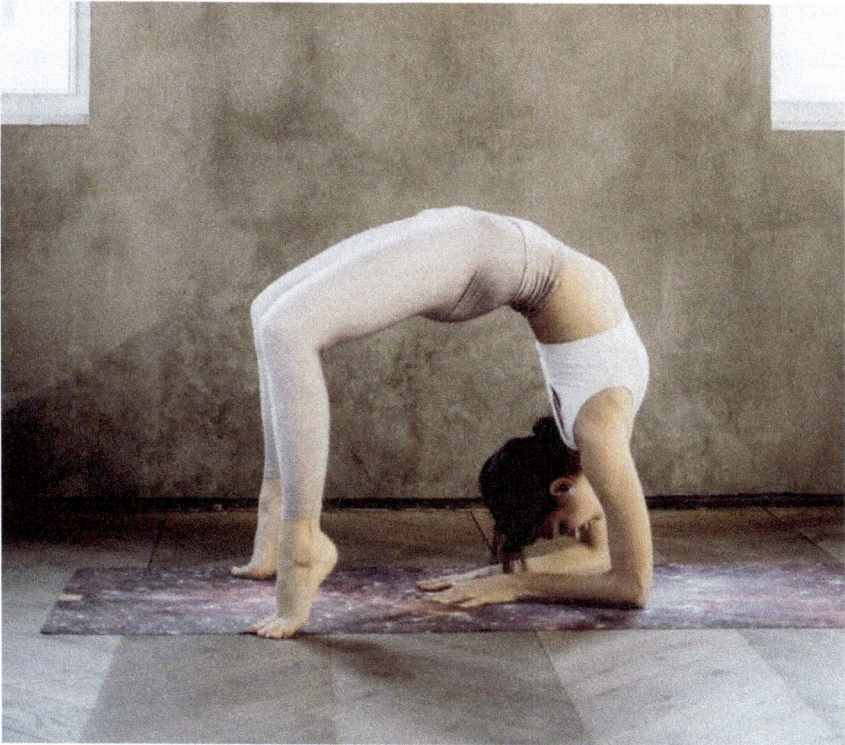

Level: Intermediate

Position: Supine

Style: Back-Bend, Stretch, Inversion, Strength, Balance

Chakra: Crown, Third Eye, Throat, Heart, Solar Plexus

Element: Thought, Light, Ether, Air, Fire

Anatomy Focus: Lower Back, Core, Chest, Neck, Psoas, Quadriceps

Begin in Corpse pose, a supine position. Bring the focus to your lower back and bend both knees placing the feet flat on the floor. Inhale and exhale and place both hands behind your head, palms on the floor. Point fingers toward the shoulders and rotate both wrists away from your body. Inhale. As you exhale, slowly lift your torso off the floor. Make sure to balance the weight of your body on both the palms of your hands as well as on the soles of both feet. Continue a normal breathing pattern as you find your comfort level. Set your gaze past your elbows in this position. Slowly lower your torso down the ground. Inhale and exhale returning to the supine position.

Warrior III

Virabhadrasana III

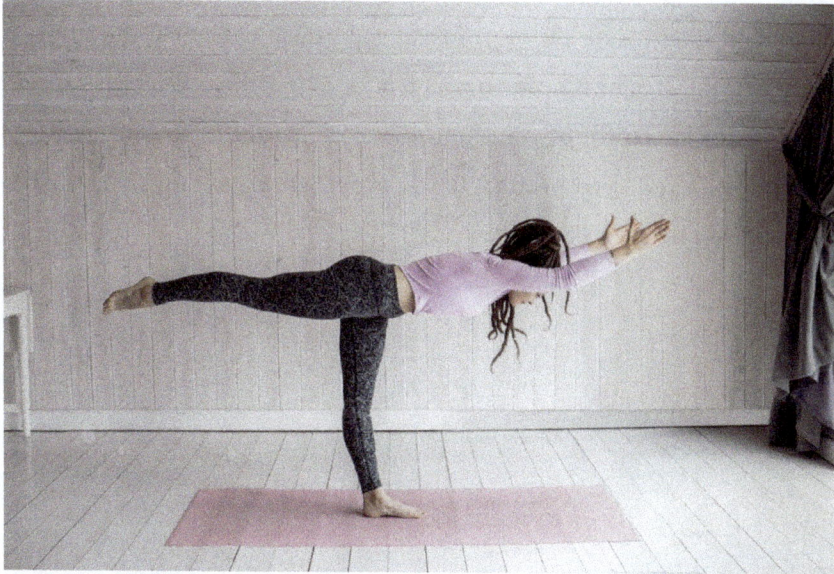

Level: Intermediate

Position: Standing

Style: Balance, Forward-Bend, Stretch, Strength, Balance

Chakra: Solar Plexus, Sacral, Root

Element: Fire, Water, Earth

Anatomy Focus: Middle Back, Core, Hamstrings, Chest, Hips, Psoas, Quadriceps

Begin in Mountain Pose. Inhale and exhale repositioning into Star Pose, feet further than hip width apart and arms raised to shoulder level. Point your palms down to the ground. Point your right foot away from the body and position your left foot facing forward. With your arms out wide, inhale and exhale tightening your core stomach muscles. Slowly shift your torso to the right, bending the right knee and placing it directly over the top of the foot. With a fluid movement, twist your upper body to the right and shift your gaze past your fingertips. Bring your left arm parallel to your right arm, palms facing one another. Twist your entire body to the right, folding your head in between your biceps and lift your left leg off the ground. Point your left foot. Inhale and exhale tightening the stomach muscles. Shift your weight as need on your left leg to find the correct balance and alignment. Point the crown of your head toward the tips of your fingers. Hold this position for a few deep breaths. Lower yyour left leg, return both arms to your side and rest back into Mountain pose.

Triangle

Trikonasana

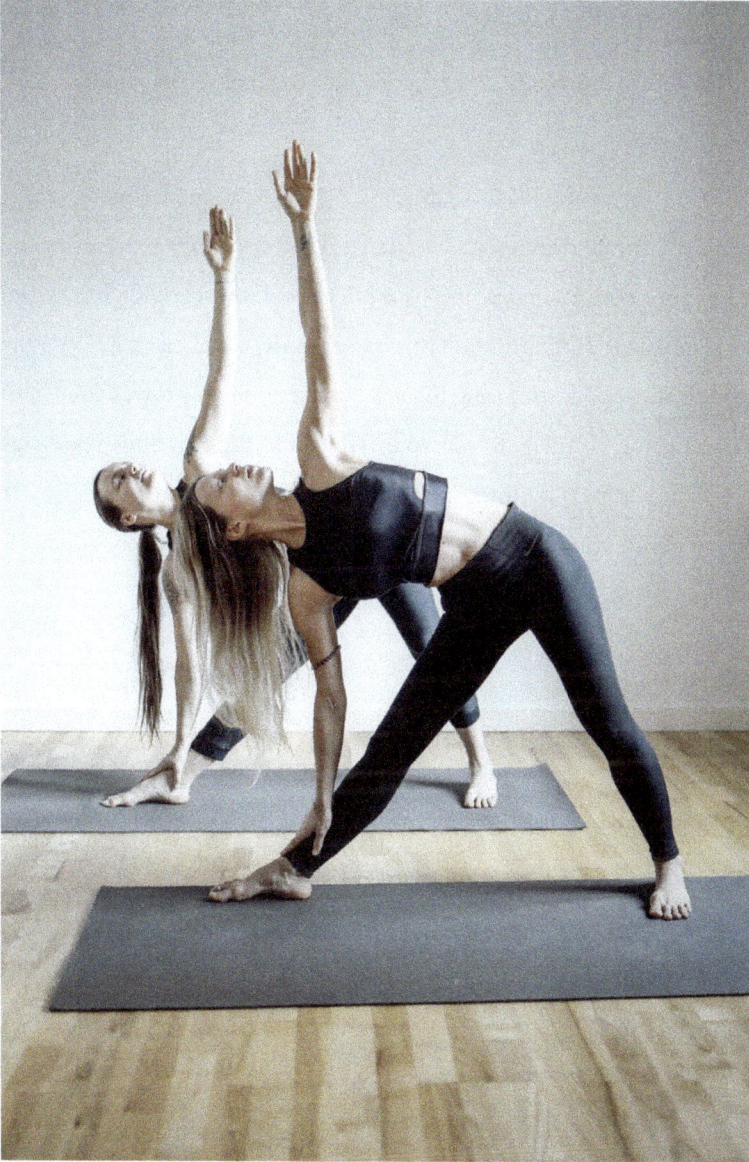

Level: Intermediate

Position: Standing

Style: Side-Bend, Stretch

Chakra: Heart, Sacral, Root

Element: Air, Water, Earth

Anatomy Focus: Arms and Shoulders, Biceps and Triceps, Core, Hamstrings, Chest, Psoas, Quadriceps

Begin in Star Pose, feet apart. Place both arms out wide, shoulder-width apart. Turn your right foot out 90 degrees and rotate your left foot forward. Inhale and exhale tightening your core and engaging your lower back muscles. Slightly rotate your lower back forward. With arms still placed out wide, slowly rotate down the right side of your body, fingers pointing toward your shin. Slowly lower your right hand to the floor behind your leg. Reach your left arm to the sky. Shift your gaze upward past your fingertips. Continue breathing through the pose. Slowly rotate back to Star Pose. Relax your arms to your sides and walk your feet together.

Plow

Halasana

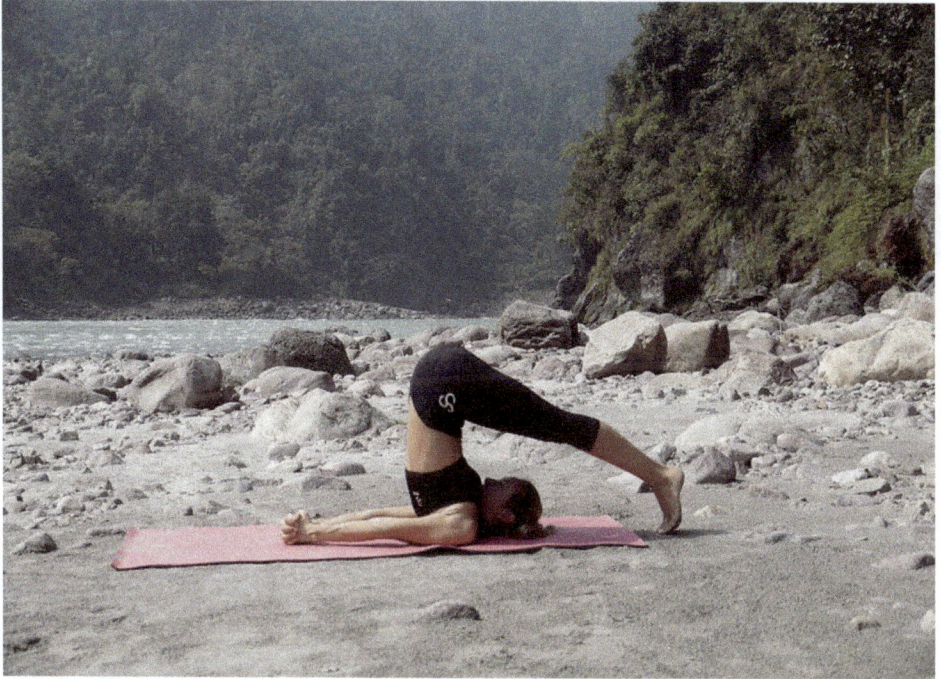

Level: Intermediate

Position: Supine

Style: Inversion, Stretch

Chakra: Crown, Third Eye, Throat, Solar Plexus

Element: Thought, Light, Ether, Fire

Anatomy Focus: Lower, Middle and Upper Back, Core, Hamstrings, Hips, Neck, Pelvic

Begin in supine position with both legs on the floor. Inhale and raise both legs to a 90 degree angle. Exhale pushing your arms and palms to the floor, rotate your legs completely over your head. Inhale and exhale as your toes touch the floor behind your head. Continue breathing through the pose. Lower both legs back to supine position.

Low Lunge

Parsva Anjaneyasana

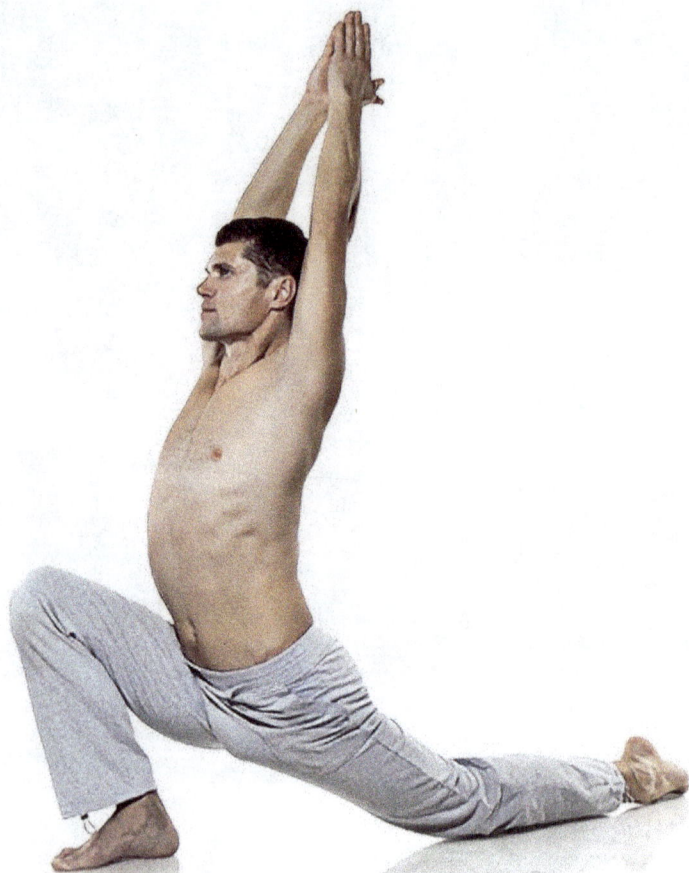

Level: Intermediate

Position: Sitting

Style: Side-Bend, Stretch, Strength, Balance

Chakra: Sacral, Root

Element: Water, Earth

Anatomy Focus: Arms and Shoulders, Upper Back, Biceps and Triceps, Core, Chest, Hips, Knees, Psoas, Quadriceps

Follow the steps from Warrior Pose II to move into a Low Lunge. Once in Warrior Pose II, raise both arms above your head and lower your right knee to the mat. Inhale and exhale resting the entire right leg straight behind your body. Let your knee rest gently on the mat. Your left knee should be directly above the top of your foot. Continue moving through the pose by lowering your shoulders and allowing your hips to drift slowly toward your mat stretching the hamstrings. If your knee begins to feel a painful pressure, place a blanket or mat underneath to add a cushion during this pose. Inhale and exhale. Move your right leg in front of your body, lower both arms and relax back into Child's Pose as needed.

Side Plank

Vasisthasana

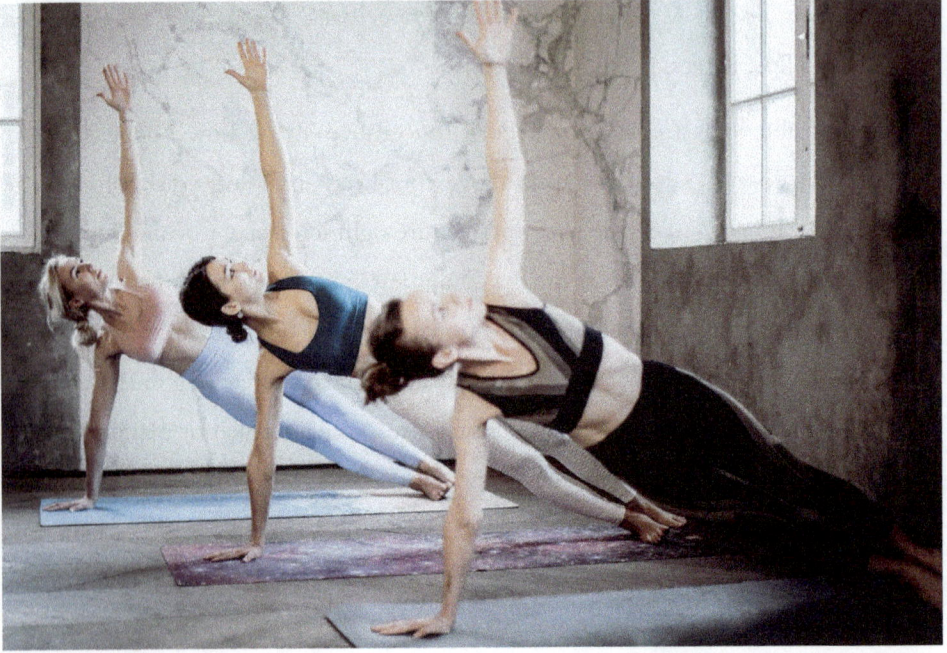

Level: Intermediate

Position: Sitting

Style: Balance, Stretch, Strength

Chakra: Solar Plexus

Element: Fire

Anatomy Focus: Arms and Shoulders, Biceps and Triceps, Core

Begin in Plank pose. Inhale and rotate your entire body to the right side. Lift your left arm to the sky and shift your gaze upward. Let your left foot rest firmly on your right foot. Push through your right palm for balance and alignment. Engage your stomach muscles to provide core support. Rotate back to Plank pose and sit back into Child's pose as needed.

Half Moon

Ardha Chandrasana

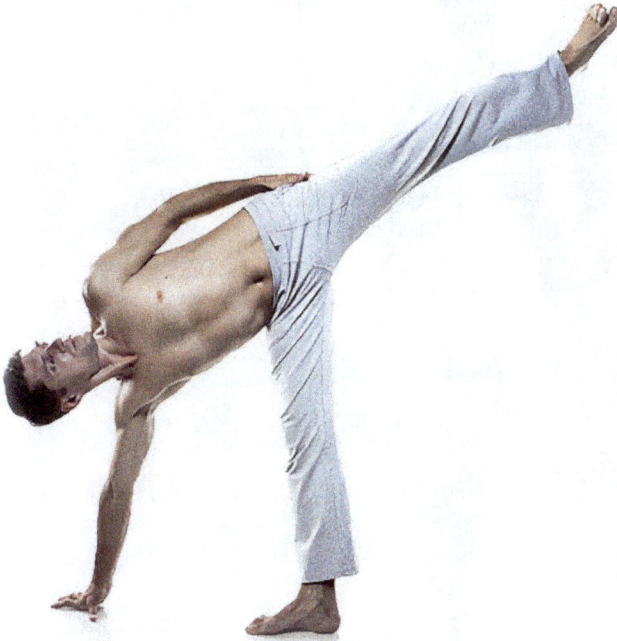

Level: Intermediate

Position: Standing

Style: Side-Bend, Inversion, Strength, Balance

Chakra: Sacral, Root

Element: Water, Earth

Anatomy Focus: Biceps and Triceps, Core, Hamstrings, Hips, Psoas, Quadriceps

Stand in Mountain Pose. Use a yoga block as needed. Place the block beside your mat within arm's reach. Spread both legs, turn your right foot to the right toward the block and point your left foot forward. Inhale and exhale and slowly lean to your right placing your right hand on the block, or on the floor. Raise your left leg so that it is parallel to your mat. Lift your left hand to the sky and shift your gaze past your fingertips. Return to Mountain Pose.

Dancer Pose

Natarajasana

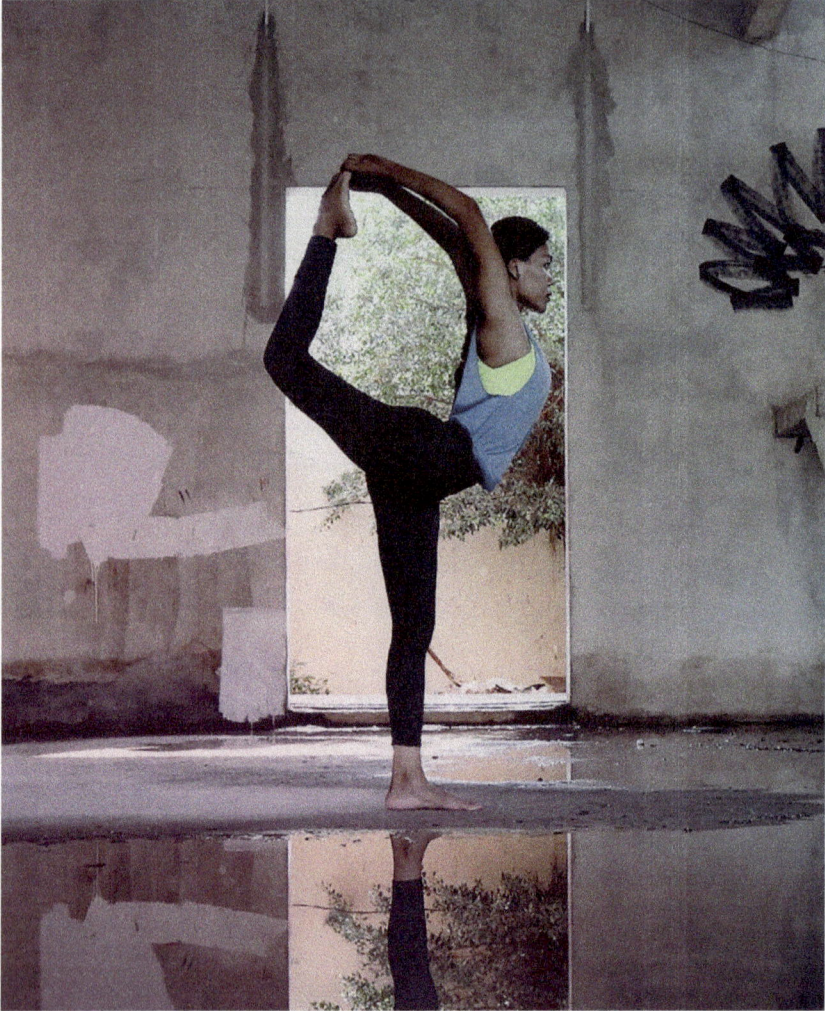

Level: Intermediate

Position: Standing

Style: Stretch, Back-Bend, Strength, Balance

Chakra: Heart, Solar-Plexus

Element: Air, Fir

Anatomy Focus: Lower Back, Biceps and Triceps, Hamstrings, Chest, Hips, Psoas, Quadriceps

Dancer Pose begins in Mountain Pose. Straighten your spine and bring your lower back slightly inward. Engage your core. Inhale and exhale bending the right knee letting the heel of your foot reach the buttocks. Stretch your right hand behind your body. Grab the toes of your right foot. Continue to inhale and exhale lifting your chest and tightening your stomach muscles. Reach your left hand straight out in front of your body. Take a deep breath in and out and twist your shoulders. Roll your fingers and thumb of your right hand around your big toe. Rotate the right elbow and shoulders allowing your arm to migrate above your head. Continue to stretch the left arm in front of you while maintaining your core balance. Plant your left foot firmly on your mat engaging the heel as well as each toe for proper balance and alignment. Slowly rotate your right arm over your head, releasing the right foot. Return to Mountain Pose.

Advanced Poses

Reclined Middle Split

Supta Trivikramasana

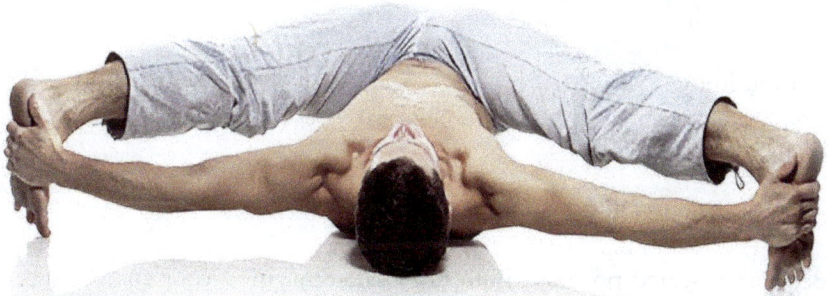

Level: Advanced

Position: Supine

Style: Stretch

Chakra: Sacral, Root

Element: Water, Earth

Anatomy Focus: Quadriceps

Begin seated in Staff Pose. Slowly roll onto your back. Inhale and exhale planting your left leg firmly on the mat. Raise your right leg to a 90 degree angle. Grasp the big right toe and rotate your right hip. Engage the stomach muscles on the exhale and bring the right knee closer to your chest. Slowly stretch the right leg closer to your shoulder loosening the hamstrings. Release the right leg down to a supine position.

Seated Middle Split

Samakonasana

Level: Advanced

Position: Sitting

Style: Stretch

Chakra: Root

Element: Earth

Anatomy Focus: Hips, Quadriceps

Begin in a seated position, Butterfly Pose. Straighten your spine. Lower both shoulders and engage your core. Inhale and exhale widening both legs to the corner of your mat. Tuck your lower back and place both hands firmly in front of you on the mat. Lower your chin to your chest and slowly roll forward supporting your upper body with both hands. Relax into the pose letting gravity assist with the fold. Inhale and exhale. Slowly roll up one vertebrae at a time back to a seated position.

Pigeon

Kapotasana

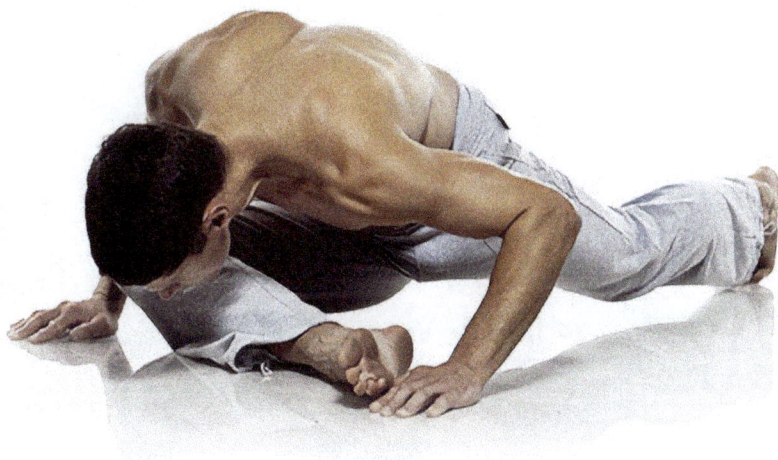

Level: Advanced

Position: Prone

Style: Stretch, Back-Bend

Chakra: Crown, Third Eye, Throat, Heart

Element: Thought, Light, Ether, Air

Anatomy Focus: Lower and Middle Back, Core, Hamstrings, Chest, Hips, Neck, Pelvic, Psoas, Quadriceps

Begin this pose in Table Top position. Bring your left knee to meet your left wrist. Inhale and lower your left hip to the floor, supporting your body with both hands on the mat. Keep your right leg straight behind your body, knee facing the floor. Lift your chest at this point for a deep stretch. Or, slowly lower your upper body over your left knee. Relax both elbows to the mat in front of you, palms down. Inhale and exhale. Push up through the palms of your hands and lift your chest of of your knees. Return to Child's pose.

Crane

Bakasana

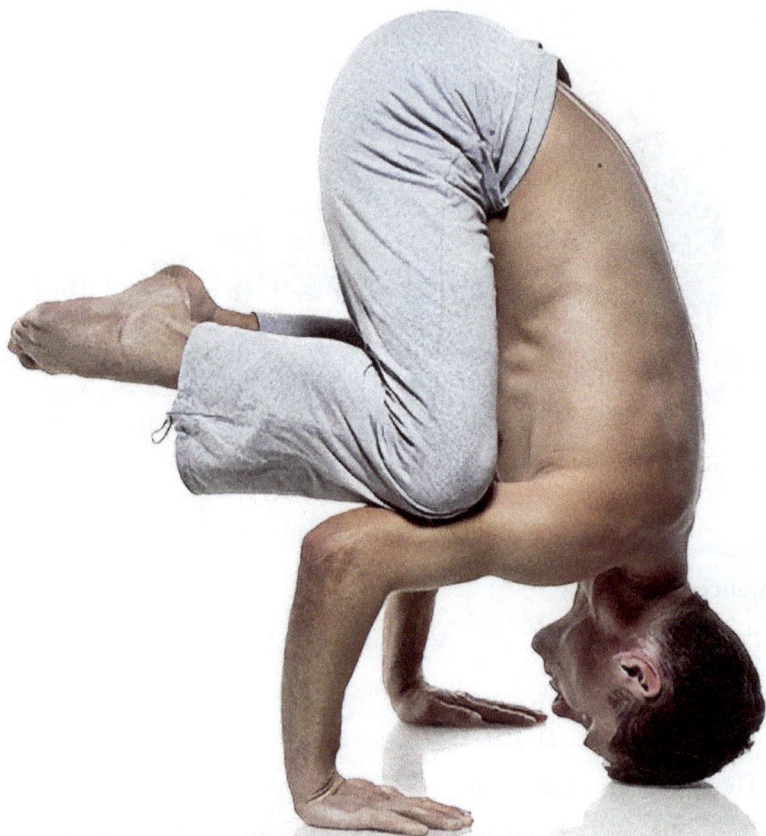

Level: Advanced

Position: Sitting

Style: Strength, Inversion, Balance

Chakra: Solar Plexus

Element: Fire

Anatomy Focus: Middle and Upper Back, Biceps and Triceps

Start this pose in a seated Garland pose. Inhale and exhale multiple times preparing for this pose. Place both palms on the floor engaging the triceps. Bring both knees to the chest and place them firmly in the armpit area. You will be on your tip toes at this point. Continue to allow a slight bend in both elbows. Take a few deep breaths. As you exhale, bend the torso forward lifted the buttocks in the air. Shift your weight onto your knees. Slowly lean forward pointing your forehead toward your mat. Allow both feet to lift off the mat while balancing your knees on top of your triceps. Inhale and exhale. Slowly roll back on to your feet and return to Garland Pose.

Headstand

Sirsasana

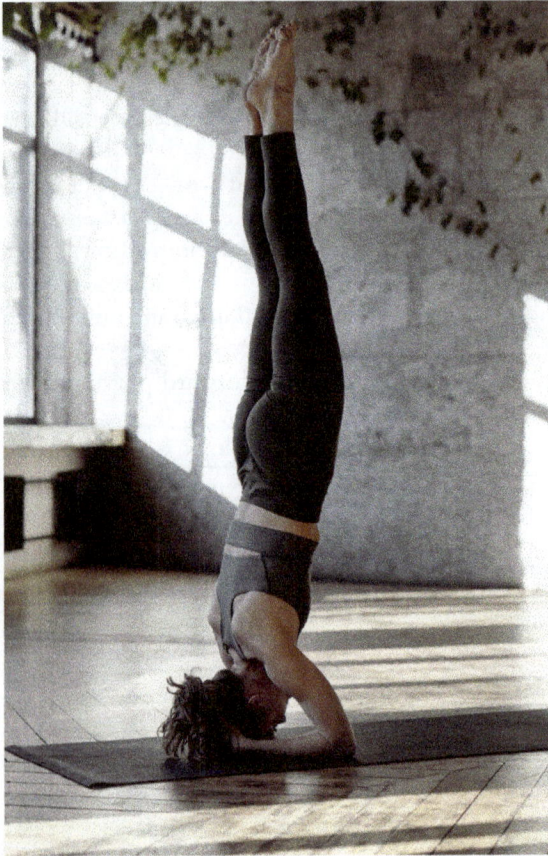

Level: Advanced

Position: Supine

Style: Inversion, Strength, Balance

Chakra: Crown, Third Eye, Throat

Element: Thought, Light, Ether

Anatomy Focus: Lower Back, Biceps and Triceps, Neck

Begin by kneeling on your mat. Rest your forearms on the mat shoulder width apart. Interlock your fingers and place the crown of your head on the mat. Cup the back of your head with your hands. After securing your head position, tuck both knees into your stomach. Inhale and exhale engaging your core and tightening the hip area. Begin to rest your weight onto your forearms and slowly lift one knee off the floor. Keep your heel close to your buttocks. Lift the opposite knee from the floor keeping both knees close to the lower body. Inhale and exhale and tightening the stomach muscles. Shift your weight off of your head and onto your elbows for balance. Slowly straighten both legs while engaging the core with every breath. Point your toes. Inhale and exhale. Gently lower one foot at a time back to a kneeling position. Slowly roll up to a final standing position.

Scorpion

Vrschikasana

Level: Advanced

Position: Prone

Style: Strength, Back-Bend, Inversion, Balance

Chakra: Crown, Third Eye, Throat

Element: Thought, Light, Ether

Anatomy Focus: Arms and Shoulders, Lower and Middle Back, Biceps and Triceps

Begin in Downward Dog. Lower both elbows down to the floor, resting both forearms on the mat. Follow the same steps as the Headstand pose to lift your feet into the air. Tuck both knees into your stomach. Inhale and exhale engaging your core and tightening the hip area. Begin to rest your weight onto your forearms and slowly lift one knee off the floor. Keep your heel close to your buttocks. Lift the opposite knee from the floor keeping both knees close to the lower body. Shift your weight onto your hands, forearms and elbows. Inhale and exhale. Slowly straighten both legs while engaging the core with every breath. Point your toes toward the sky. Inhale and exhale tightening the stomach muscles. Slowly begin to bend both knees. Point the toes toward the back of your head. Bend from the middle to upper back. Gently begin to lower one leg at a time back down to the mat. Relax back into Child's Pose.

PART III

Your Restorative Practice

Restorative Yoga is a calming practice. A practice that many of us need daily.

This specific type of yoga helps to release tension, anxiety and stress that stems from busy daily activities, traumatic circumstance or life-changing events. Restorative yoga typically utilizes props including blankets, bolsters, blocks, aromatherapy, etc. Props in restorative yoga assist with body alignment, relaxation and weight balance. They can also aide in alleviating pressure in certain areas of the body while practicing asanas.

Most of us are aware of the popular yoga classes that incorporate constant movement and active poses. Restorative yoga, however, utilizes the poses that allow your body to slowly stretch in to a relaxed state. Breathing techniques and meditation are incorporated into each pose prompting the body to slow down and enter a mode of stillness. These restorative poses and techniques ease symptoms related to anxiety, depression, stress, pain and trauma-related injuries.

The main ingredient in restorative yoga is time and patience. Each pose is held for a longer period of time allowing the body to enter into a state of mind-body unification. Holding the poses for a longer period of time also provides a deeper stretch, "stretching to the bone," as some would explain.

Daily life can send us reeling through a multitude of emotions. Simply going to the grocery store can ingnite a high level of stress. Unexpected, life-altering events may bring about intense changes affecting the way we react to certain situations. The way we handle stressful situations can cause the physical body to remain tense with no sign of relief. The human body is capable of leading a very active life. We must take the time to give our minds and our bodies a break. If we do not, our immune system might deteriorate, and our minds will fade.

So, when do we slow down?

More importantly, how do we slow down? Once that roller coaster called life starts chugging away, most of us don't know how to stop, or how to slow down. We need some kind of assistance or daily practice that will help us to decompress. We must stop running ourselves into the ground.

Learning how to recognize a quiet moment, a peaceful place, the sound of silence – We all long for each of those opportunities, but refuse to stop and realize that they are most likely right in front of our faces. Stillness is very important. And, the older we get, the harder it is to return to that state of stillness.

Generally speaking, yoga is defined as the unification of the mind and body. It is the practice of harmonizing the physical body with the spiritual body and returning to a conscious state of stillness and mindfulness.

When practicing the restorative method of yoga, time is a very important aspect. In restorative yoga, you will hold the asanas for 3-5x longer than in other yoga practices. Typically, in one restorative yoga session, you may only complete 3-5 poses. As opposed to an active yoga session, you may flow continuously through 10-20 poses.

Some examples of restorative yoga poses are Child's pose, Corpse pose, Legs-Up-The-Wall pose, etc. During each pose, you can incorporate very specific breathing techniques and meditation methods. Holding the poses for a longer period of time also allows you to adjust your body for proper alignment and balance.

Let's face it, we are all uniquely built. Not one of us is the same, physically, emotionally or mentally. Therefore, we must adjust our yoga practice to fit our own personal needs.

There are many ways to create your own unique restorative yoga practice.

Yoga is for Everyone

First of all, let's get one thing straight. You do not have to be perfect to practice any type of yoga. Yoga is a balancing of the mind and the body. We all have very unique body types. No one is made the same. Your yoga practice is exactly just that - a practice tailored to fit the needs of your mind and your body.

You may feel

 like you are overweight, too tall, too short, not flexible, too skinny, etc. Try to let go of whatever inhibitions may be keeping you from jumping into your first routine. Many people immediately associate the word yoga with headstands and pretzel poses. While those advanced activities are certainly a piece of the yoga puzzle, they do not define yoga.

For example, let's say you have had a really rough day at the office, or with the kiddos. Maybe you are dealing with a loss in the family or financial struggles. Maybe your day, week, month or year just hasn't gone as planned. If you know the basics of yoga and how to practice on your own, you just may be able to ease that anxiety or calm the stress that comes during those difficult times.

But, hey! Maybe you are having a great day, week, month or year. That sounds wonderful, doesn't it? Then let your yoga practice serve that cherry on top. Learning the simple art of taking breaths throughout your day and mastering the act of sitting still could totally change your life.

There's nothing wrong with feeling shy at first when it comes to deciding to start your own yoga practice. But, remember, you are important and need to be healthy and happy. Taking that first step toward the local yoga studio or even just setting up a yoga mat at home could be one of the best steps of your life!

A Restorative Practice at Home

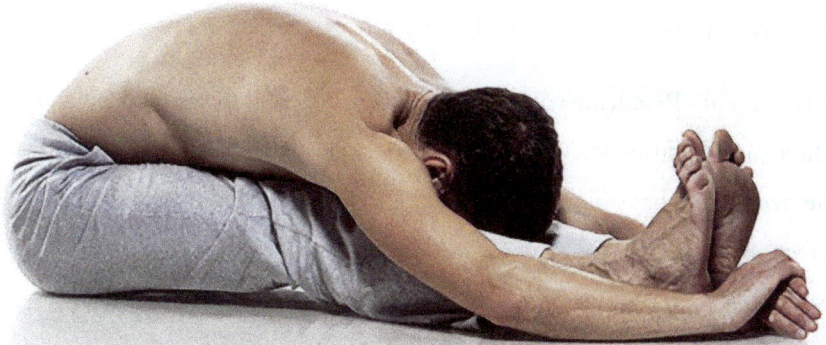

Restorative Yoga can absolutely be practiced at home.

Gyms and studios are fabulous practice areas as well. But, there may be days where you can't make it out of the house. Or, your schedule isn't permitting a quick run to the gym. Sometimes yoga studios have to reorganize their classes and you usual time slot isn't available anymore.

That's ok!

Let's create our own home studio for those days.

Follow these simple steps to begin setting up your own home practice.

1. Find a Quiet Spot - Find a space in your home away from loud noises and people. That space may be in a quiet room, in the backyard, or any peaceful spot that you choose.

2. Set the Mood - Once you have found the perfect space, dim the lights, lower the shades and turn down any loud sounds. If you enjoy a favorite scent, turn on an oil diffuser, light a candle, or burn incense.

3. Create Space - Yoga requires space. Once your yoga mat is situated, make sure to move any objects that may get in the way of your arms and legs.

4. Be Patient - Practicing yoga at home is very different than practicing in a studio. There may be times when you have to check on the kids, answer the door, check the oven, etc. That's ok. Simply deciding to begin yoga is a huge step in the right direction.

Breathing Techniques

Each yoga pose should include a breathing pattern, or breathing technique if you will. There are many types of breathing patterns to follow. It is perfectly acceptable to create a breathing pace that works best for your practice.

Let's face it, we all lack the proper amount of oxygen. We readily give in to the ease of shallow breathing throughout our busy day, and we forget to take in those absolutely necessary deep breaths.

The practice of breathing in yoga is called Pranayama.

If yoga does nothing other than prompt us to breath for an hour, then so be it. In fact, if you are a beginner yoga student, simply just learning how to breath may be the extent of your first few classes. Enjoy it, because the hard poses come next!

Practicing how to breath seems like a simple task. Just wait though. This involuntary act of breathing that we so recklessly abandon too much in a day may give you that energy boost you've been looking for. And, guess what? You can practice breathing anywhere!

So, let's breath.

Pursed Lip Breathing

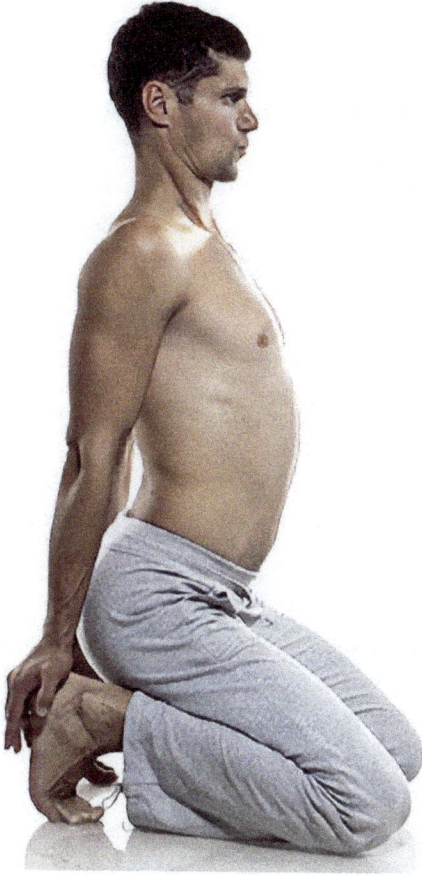

1. Sit quietly and relax your neck and shoulders. Place your arms beside your body and let your hands lay on your lap or mat.

2. Inhale through your nose and hold for two counts.

3. Purse your lips as if you were drinking through a straw.

4. Gently blow your entire breath out through your lips until your abdomen releases completely.

Diaphragm Breathing

1. Lie on your back in a quiet space. You can bend your knees for comfort or simply rest both legs on the floor.

2. Place one hand on your chest and the other hand on your stomach.

3. Inhale through your nose allowing your belly to extend.

4. Exhale through your pursed lips, feeling your belly empty all of its air, releasing down into your spine.

Lion's Breathing

1. Sit comfortably in a quiet space with legs crossed and hands placed on both knees.

2. Inhale through your nose letting your chest expand. Lower both shoulders.

3. Open your mouth wide and exhale making the "Ha" sound until you've expended all of the air in your belly.

Alternate Nostril Breathing

1. Begin in a seated position

2. Lift your hand to your nose. Press your pointer and middle finger down against your palm and release the index and pinky fingers toward the sky.

3. Press your thumb against your right nostril. Closing the airway.

4. Inhale through your left nostril.

5. Release the thumb and exhale through your right nostril.

6. Repeat on the other side.

Coherent Breathing

1. Find a comfortable seated position

2. Inhale for 5 counts.

3. Exhale for 5 counts.

Any one of these breathing techniques can be performed during your restorative yoga practice. The beauty behind the art of breathing is that it can be done anywhere, preferably in a quiet and calm space.

There are, however, many times during the day where you are not able to find a quiet space. Let's say you begin to feel anxious during an important business meeting. You could quietly begin the "Coherent Breathing" technique without causing a scene.

Not only can you practice these breathing steps during a restorative yoga session, but you can also apply them in everyday situations.

Meditation Methods

Meditatiion in an intergral piece to every type of yoga practice. In fact, meditation should be an important part of each person's daily routine. There is no one way to meditate. Personal meditation practices are based each person's unique character, specific surroundings and life experiences.

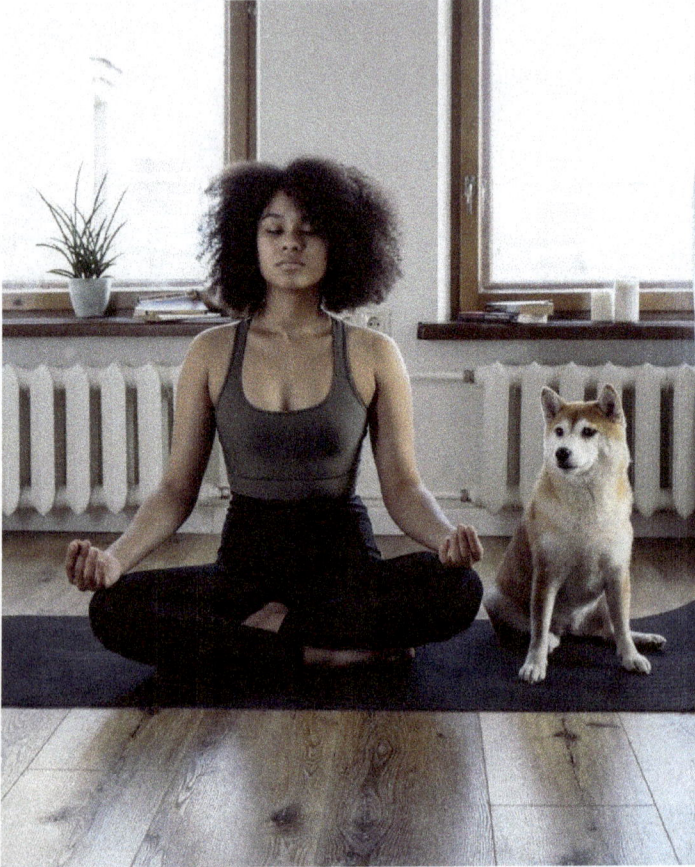

There are hundreds of meditation techniques spanning many different cultures, religions and spiritual practices. Choosing a meditation method that is right for you may take time. It is important to find the right space – space where you feel comfortable enough to be yourself.

Meditation is your personal piece of art. Your thoughts during meditation are your own and belong to no one else. It is a time for you to be honest with yourself. This is your space to approach the places in your mind that are typically suppressed in real life.

There are two types of meditation – guided and unguided.

Guided meditation is exactly as it sounds. A teacher helps to guide you through the steps of a particular meditation practice. The teacher explains how the mind operates, walks you through step-by-step and assists in implementing the meditation into your daily life.

Unguided meditation simply involves one person – You. This method of meditation allows you to decide exactly where, when and how you want to practice. You are the teacher when it comes to an unguided meditation practice.

Simply put, meditation teaches focus. Our day-to-day lives are constantly filled with messages, ads, phone calls, texts, requests, deadlines, etc. Our brain never gets a moment to itself. Meditation is the art of finally stopping all the ruckus in your head and giving your personal thoughts some much needed attention.

As we continue to deal with all of these distractions, our mind becomes adept to wandering. We never get the chance to complete our thoughts. We are constantly distracted.

Meditation teaches us how to recognize when our mind begins to wander away from the initial thought. As you practice mindfulness in meditation, you learn how to bring your thoughts back to consciousness and awareness.

In restorative yoga, meditation can be used to create stillness while practicing the asanas. It helps to counteract distractions, anxious feelings, social awkwardness and negative energy.

Meditation during each restoratice yoga pose engages the mind-body unification practice that defines yoga as a whole.

Alignment and Balance – Props

Props are very important in restorative yoga. Yoga props assist physically in reaching your yoga goals. By utilizing props in your yoga practice, you are less likely to say, "I can't!"

We've all said or heard the "I can't do it" comments when it comes to yoga.

"I'm just not that flexible."

"I can't do yoga because I'm overweight."

"I'm too old."

"I had surgery years ago and just can't move the way I used to."

The best response to anyone justifying there inability to practice yoga is, "YES! You can."

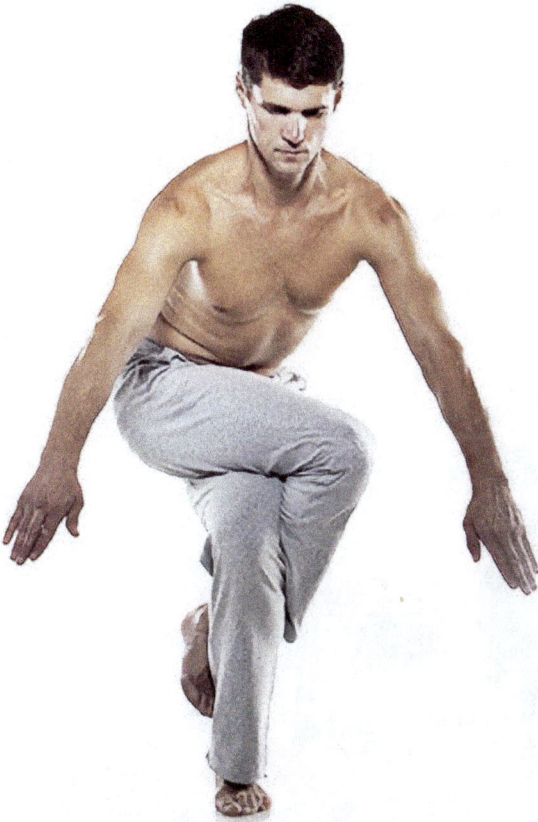

Yoga isn't about practicing like everyone else. Yoga isn't about looking like the girl or guy online or in the health and fitness books.

Yoga is simply practicing like YOU practice.

There is no one human body made exactly like the other. Your hand may not reach the floor during the Side Angle pose. That's ok! You may need a yoga block under your neck during Savasana to ease your lower back pain. Maybe rolling a blanket and placing it under you knees for spine support is necessary. There is no right or wrong way to practice yoga. It's all ok!

Everyone is different.

You are unique and so shall your yoga practice be!

Restorative yoga incorporates many different props that hav different responsibilities. They are there to aide your body's alignment and balance as your move through each pose.

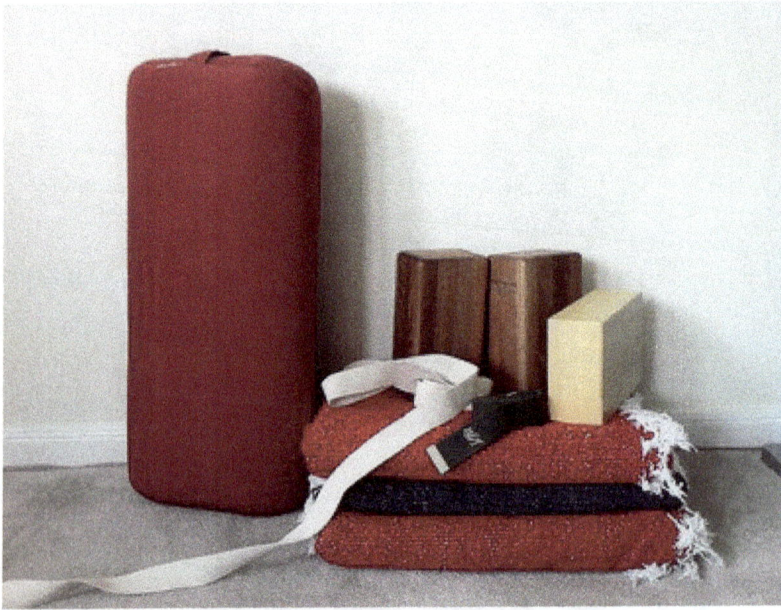

One important thing to remember when adding a prop to your pose, be patient. We may feel like we need to rush to grab a prop before trying a new pose. It's not important how quickly you get into the pose. Take your time. Listen first as the teacher explains the elements of the pose. Then decide whether or not you will need a prop based on how your body reacts to each movement.

If you need to come out of the pose to grab a prop, then do so. If your neck is straining, don't throw your shoulder out trying to reach the block or the blanket.

Be patient with your body. Utilizing a prop should create physical and mental relaxation, not added stress.

So, what in the world are these "props" we keep mentioning. Ok, let's see what all of these crazy blocks, straps and bolsters are all about!

Blocks

Yoga blocks are made of wood, foam or cork. These blocks can support your body in many of the yoga poses. For example, you can place the block next to you during a Side Angle or Triangle pose. This allows your to place your hand on the block instead of the floor. A block can also be used as a head rest during Savasana or under your lower back during Bridge pose.

Bolster

The bolster prop is most widely used in restorative yoga. This is a reactangular cushion providing support for many heart-opening and lower back exercises. The bolster can be used under the forehead during Child's pose or under the knees in Tree Top pose.

Straps

Straps are like large rubber bands used in many "stretch" poses. They act as extensions of the arm or leg for poses such as the Dancer pose or the Wheel pose. Straps can be used during a forward fold by wrapping it around your wrists and feet assisting in the stretch.

Sandbags

Sandbags are like large bean bags used to add weight on the body for a deeper stretch. They can be used on the hips during poses such as the Supine Twist

Blanket

Blankets in yoga have many different uses. You can use a blanket as your practice mat, folded as a cushion for an elbow or a knee, or as a pillow for your head during restorative poses.

Eye Pillow

The yoga eye pillow is used to block out light and helps to calm the brain. It facilitates a deeper meditation and filter out visual distractions. It is perfect for Savasana and can sometime be scented for aromatherapy.

Mat

The yoga mat is where it all happens. Your mat can be most anything that feels comfortable to you. Some use the typical foam mat that rolls up and is easy to carry. Some yoga students like to use blankets, or a"serape." Just make sure that whatever you choose offers support, stability and comfort.

Essential Oils

Aromatherapy changes the game! There's certainly nothing wrong with a little sweat during your yoga practice. But, when it's time to relax and soothe, choosing the right essential oil scent is important. Scents such as lavender, jasmine, sage, lemongrass and vanilla are all very popular in the restorative yoga practice.

Music

Set the tone with relaxing tunes. In a world of digital downloads, it's simple and easy to add music as you flow through each restorative yoga pose.

Yoga Flow

Flow yoga is a term that relates to a style of yoga focusing on patterned breathing and rhythmic movement.

Flowing through yoga is a beautiful movement. There are thousands of poses and many different sequences. That's why choosing your favorite type of yoga is a good decision. You can focus on practicing and developing the seqences or "flow" that works best for you and your body.

Yoga flow teach the body and the mind to work harmoniously together. Not only are you placing your body into specific poses, but your mind is learning to transition through to the next pose. This requires a reorganization of the mind, giving the brain a mental boost. Practicing continuous physical movement changes our thought patterns.. It helps us to get out of a rut sometimes. It also helps to boost our energy by bring on new challenges. When we train our brain to reorganize, we create a wealth of new thoughts and ideas.

Increasing mental focus and training our bodies to become stronger and more agile is very important at any age in life. Yoga flow is a low impact method used to gain strength of the mind and the body. The series of poses in a "flow" exercise, utilizes rhythmic breathing. It's very important to calculate each movement and whether or not you should be inhaling or exhaling at the same time. Your breath pattern is used to measure how long you will hold the pose. It also helps us to count through each movements during the same pose.

The process of patterned breathing while moving through a yoga sequence has many physical benefits. Breathing patterns can stabilize your heart rate, regulate body temperature and help you to maintain consistent movement all the way to the end of the exercise. Synchronizing your breath stables your heart rate and assists your body in releasing a balanced amount of heat. Therefore, your muscles will stretch and loosen properly during each exercise.

Learning yoga flow can be easy. The most important first step is to sign up for a class taught by a certified or qualified yoga instructor. It may be a good idea to initially choose a smaller class, especially if you are a true beginner in the yoga world. This way the instructor will have the time to address each student on a more personal level. He or she will have the chance to monitor your movemements. They can also personally assist you in modifying the pose based on your ability.

Attending a smaller class will also give you the opportunity to assess the space. Where should you place your mat? How much space will you need? Where are the props? Yoga flow classes also require intense focus. A smaller class can lessen the stress of unwanted distractions such as cramped space, the lack of props, phone noises, foot traffic, etc.

Obviously, the poses that you can expect in your Yoga Flow class depend on the level of the class.

Yoga levels are pretty basic – Beginner, Intermediate and Advanced. The instructor will most likely progress through a series of the same poses over a certain period of clases. Make sure to inquire about which level that you will be signing up for. There may be certain poses, positions, bends, stretches, etc. that could cause injury if you are not ready. This is true especially for back bends and inversion poses.

Yoga is a process. Everything you learn in your beginner class sets the foundation for your practice in the intermediate and advanced classes. So, sign up for that beginner class and plan to perfect the easy poses.

Your body will thank you.

The Many Types of Yoga

Hatha

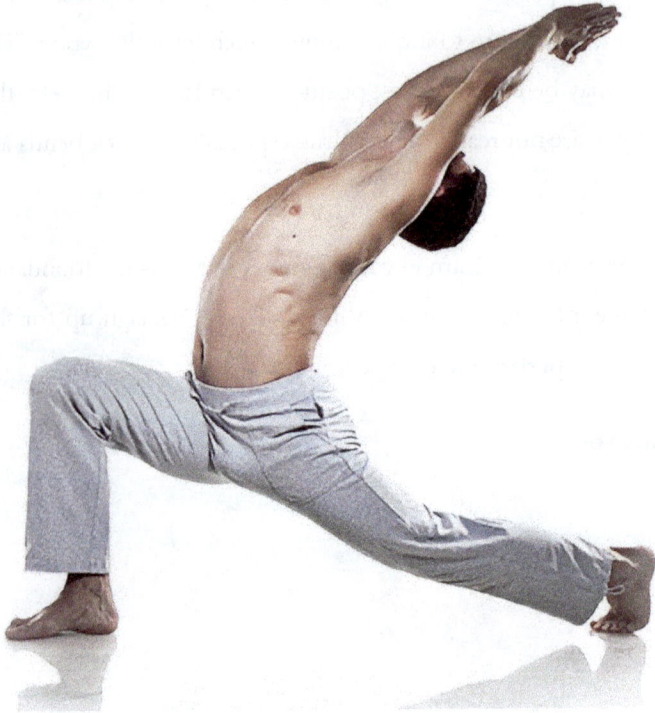

Hatha is the yoga practice that specifically deals with physical poses. Hatha is very common in Western culture. When people think of yoga, the physical poses immediately come to mind.

Hatha poses are slower and the movements are very calming. Yoga flow is integrated into a Hatha practice.

Also though the poses are slower and more relaxed, your body and mind still benefit from the poses. By flowing through the poses at a more relaxed pace, you can also focus on your breathing techniques and alignment during each movement. Hatha is a great practice for beginners.

Iyengar

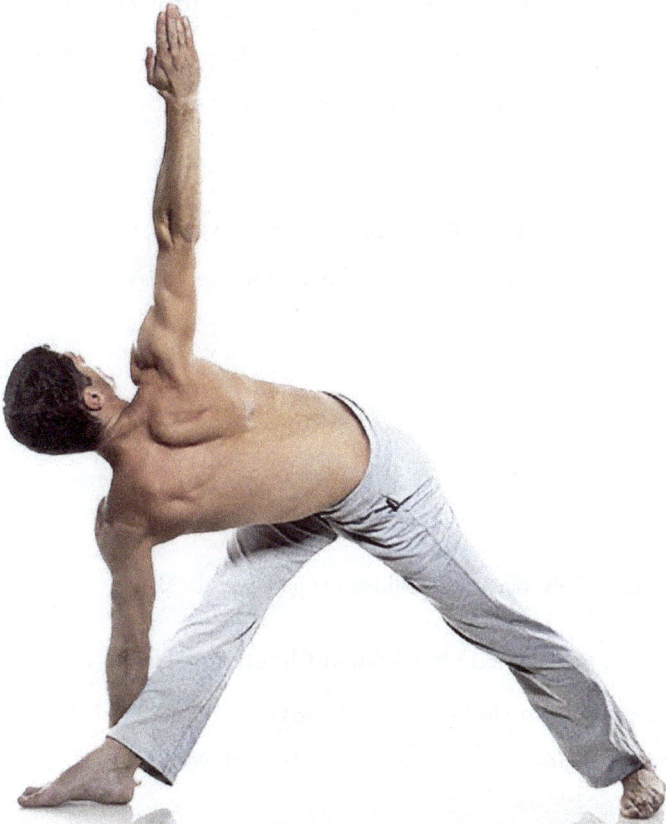

Iyengar was the man's name who founded Iyengar yoga. He was a very influential teacher in the yoga community.

Proper alignment and balance are the focus in Iyengar yoga. Poses are held for longer periods of time. Props such as mats, blocks and straps etc. are typically used in this practice. Poses are also be held longer in Hatha. Holding the poses for a longer period of time allow for a deeper stretch in order to promote the elongation of the muscles.

Iyengar promotes wellness of the mind and strong focus when moving into each pose. If you are dealing with an injury, this yoga practice allows you to pinpoint that specific area of your body to promote healing. And Iyengar instructor teaches the many aspects of each pose. He or she may note how each movement benefits a specific muscle.

You probably won't break a sweat during an Iyengar class either. Instead, each practice should end with mental clarity and relaxed muscles.

Bikram

You will definitely sweat in a Bikram yoga style class!

Bikram yoga was named after Bikram Choudhury. He developed this yoga style by turning the heat up in the room during class. Sometimes people refer to Bikram as "hot yoga." However, they are two different types of yoga.

Bikram yoga practices the same 26 poses in every class. You will practice those poses over and over again, learning and perfecting each one. The purpose of Bikram yoga is to loosen the muscles by working in a heated atmosphere.

If you plan to attend a Bikram yoga class, consult your instructor if you have been diagnosed with any ailment or sickness. You may need to modify the routine or take short breaks if you begin to feel short of breath or neasous. The temperature in a Bikram class can reach up to 104 degrees. Drink a lot of water, bring a towel and wear clothes that can withstand a heavy amount of sweat.

Ashtanga

K. Pattabhi Jois. brought Ashtanga yoga into the Western culture in the 1970's.

Ashtanga yoga focuses on consistent breathing and movement. This practice teaches you to connect a breathing pattern to the sequence of poses as directed by the instructor. It's purpose is continuous movement while following a very strenuous pace during the poses.

The yoga sequence is the same in each class. It's recommended to sign up for a few beginner classes before committing to an Ashtanga class. This way, you will become more familiar with the simple poses so that you can implement the more difficult poses during each sequence. Ashtanga yoga is designed to keep you moving.

Vinyasa

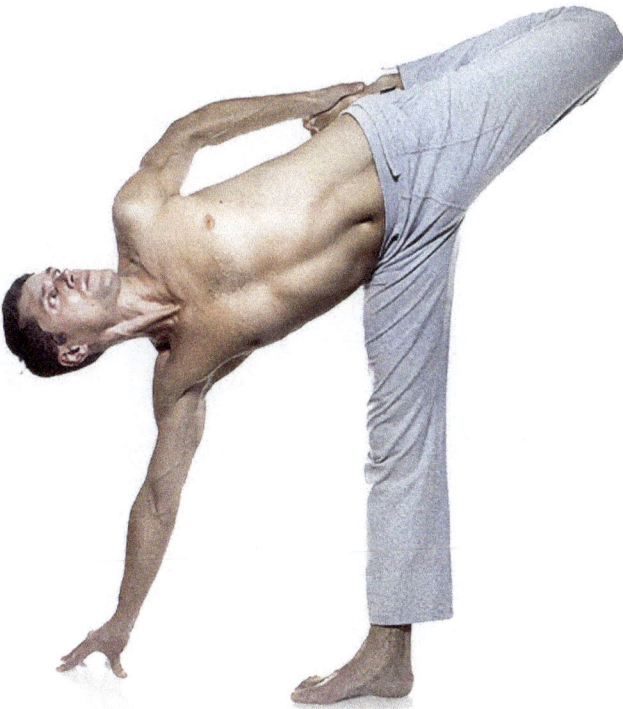

Vinyasa means to "place something in a special way."

Vinyasa is very similar to Restorative and Ashtanga yoga. The poses are held for a longer period of time. You are given more time to spend placing your body into the correct posture. With each breath, you are able to correct your alignment and balance.

Vinyasa incorporates yoga flow. While each pose is held for a longer period of time, you will still move continuously into the next pose. Depending on the instructor, the poses will most likely change with each class.

Focus is very important in a Vinyasa class. You will need to watch the instructor intently to make sure you are moving correctly into the next position. Although the pace may be slow, it is certainly continuous and can be energized with music.

Yin

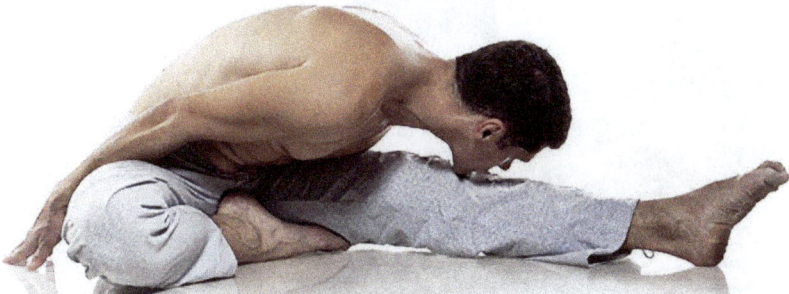

Yin is a great class for beginners. In a Yin class, you are given ample amount of time to perfect the poses for proper alignment and balance. You are also in a seated position to hold the poses for 2-5 minutes or more. It's not uncommon in a Yin class to complete only 3-5 poses within an hour. By holding the poses, Yin provides a "stretch to the bone."

This type of stretch not only stretches the muscles, but also loosens and releases the deep connective tissues. These stretch methods provide deeply relaxed muscles by the end of the class.

Meditation is also heavily integrated into a Yin practice. Since it is a slow-paced and quiet atmosphere, the student can integrate meditation into each pose.

Props are utilized in a Yin class as well. Props such as straps and blocks act as extensions of the limbs and provide a deeper stretch. This improves flexibility over time.

Restorative

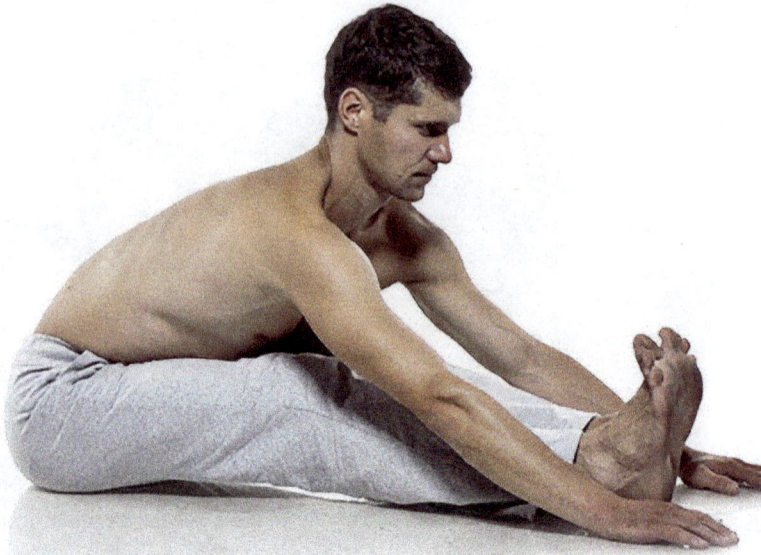

Ah, Restorative yoga. This level of a yoga practice is typically forgotten, especially in Western culture. We live in a "go-go-go" world and rarely get the option or the ability to slow down.

Most yoga classes will twist and turn your body into those pretzel poses as seen in the books and online. Not Restorative yoga. Restorative-style yoga relaxes and loosens your muscles. This practive gives you the chance to slow down and enter into a peaceful and calm mode of true rest.

Restorative yoga is best practiced in a dark, noiseless and open space. Find space that invites positive feelings and relaxing vibes. Whether your are signing up for a class at the gym or practicing at home, choose the best time of day that works for you. Obviously, make sure that you feel safe in the environment and void of any distractions. Your restorative space should be free of loud noises, cell phones tings and pings and negative energy.

Each pose in restorative yoga session should be used to relax your body. Everyone's body is different. Therefore, your restorative yoga practice should be designed to best fit the way that your body moves and stretches.

Restorative yoga poses are based heavily on props for support. These props assist each part of the body as needed. Extra blankets can cushion areas with added pressure. Bolsters aide in aligning the body and relieving painful stretchs. Straps act as extensions of the arms and legs allowing you to fasten the pose. Blocks support the neck, the back and the knees. Block can also act as landing pieces for hands and feet. You can add as many blankets as needed, folded or unfolded, to support any part of the body.

The great thing about restorative yoga is that you have time! Time to move into the position that feels best for you and your body. You have time to position a prop under, around or on top of your body for comfort.

Restorative is all about support. If your hand is dangling, or if your back is straining, grab a prop. Create your own support with the blocks, bolsters, blankets, etc. If your muscles are strained, they probably aren't being given proper support to ease into the restorative position.

Many times, this type of yoga calls for a very warm atmosphere. Some instructors will even lead you to grab an extra blanket for full body cover. Adding a weighted blanket to your body not only assists gravity in executing the pose, it also generates warmth for you're your muscles. The warmer your muscles are, the safer the stretch becomes.

Socks are also a good idea when practicing restorative yoga. In other yoga classes, you are usually instructed to practice with bare feet. However, in restorative yoga, as mentioned above, warmth is essential. Covering your feet in some form or fashion stops the release of body heat through the toes.

And, here's the kicker. You may fall asleep in a restorative yoga class. The goal is to not fall asleep. But, let's face it – warm air, relaxed muscles, blankets and a quiet room just might do the trick. It's ok. Your instructor will help to wake you properly and safely.

PART IV

<u>Energy Healing</u>

The Role of Energy in Holistic Health and Healing

Chapter 1: Energy Healing- The Key to Holistic Health

Understanding the impacts of energy imbalances and corresponding physical, mental, spiritual health

How many times have you, or another adult in your life, said the words "I just don't have the energy I used to have."? Most adults know the feeling of looking at the energy children have as they run about, enjoying life, exploring their surroundings, and never seeming to grow tired. Many of us are left reflecting back on the distant past when we, too, had such energy and wondering where it went.

From the time children enter school, they begin to be presented with expectations. Stand in a straight line, raise your hand, don't talk while the teacher is talking. Each year, the level of responsibility and expectation seems to increase. While rules, regulations, and individual responsibility are important for a functioning society, there are numerous expectations and social pressures put on people as they grow, which can be incredibly harmful.

It is generally around middle school when children become more acutely aware of their bodies and societal beauty standards, which tell them what they "should" look like. Children are likely to become aware of the trends, such as which clothes the "cool kids" are wearing. The endless battle to feel like enough begins, and can lead to a plethora of issues with self-esteem, eating disorders, and mental illness. In addition to the basic societal pressures to be accepted and considered attractive, many children are also faced with difficult situations at home where their own needs are not being met, they are having to provide for and protect themselves in the only ways they know how, avoid abusive parents, care for younger siblings, or worry about if they'll have anything to eat that day. Even if children have a relatively healthy home life, this is the age when they will begin to become aware of the issues that plague their family (every family has issues) whether this is divorce, an alcoholic parent, the death of a pet or loved one, etc.

We live in a society that thrives off of consumerism. We are flooded with images of how the next vacation, new pair of shoes, nicer car, nicer house, or perfect partner will make us happy, and all of the things we need to change about ourselves in order to fulfill those things. Eventually, all the energy we had as a child starts going towards maintaining our image in society, trying to have all the "best" life has to offer (which always happens to be everything we do not have), and attempting to be as "successful" as possible in the eyes of society and other people. With no time to rest in the present moment, recharge, and appreciate what we already have, it is no wonder, so many of us are completely drained of energy. In such a fast-paced society that discourages breaks, our energy will become depleted, and we will find ourselves thrown out of balance and unable to obtain true happiness and well-being. Over time, this depletion and imbalance can lead to a sense of spiritual disconnection, extreme mental health issues, and an increased risk of physical pain, illness, and even earlier death.

Chapter 2: Energy Healing and Overcoming Suffering

Energy and Grief/Trauma

Every human being knows that loss is a natural part of life. The one certain thing in life is that we, and everyone we know, is going to die. However, in such a fast-paced society, we are often given a very short grace period before being expected to swallow our grief and "move on" when we lose those closest to us. It is not abnormal for people to receive a bereavement period of only a few days before being expected to be back in the classroom or office and be fully functional. There is very little space for the grief journey, and most people are expected to harbor their feelings and keep their grief to themselves.

The grief process is expansive and incredibly energy draining. When we don't receive the adequate support from those around us, or adequate space to heal, our body begins to break down piece by piece. The empty spaces within us will swallow us up into states of depression, numbness, isolation, and pure exhaustion. Just like a wound being denied the correct treatment and care, the wounds of unresolved grief will fester and leave us feeling completely drained of energy and vitality for life.

Unresolved trauma also has an incredibly destructive impact on the body. Trauma can occur as a result of grief itself, as well as emotional or domestic abuse, accident or illness, war, sexual assault, childhood maltreatment, etc. The body holds trauma in various places, and the brain switches over from the logical ability to discern safety and danger into an easily triggered emotional state. An overactive emotional brain loses the ability to think clearly, make decisions, and recognize threats. People who have unresolved trauma are likely to be easily triggered and deal with unexplained outbursts of anger, fear, relationship issues, reckless behavior, and health problems. When trauma sits in the body unresolved, the brain is unable to understand that the traumatic event has ended. Therefore, it will stay in a consistent fight-or-flight state, which is incredibly draining and will leave the body with no energy. Not only will trauma victims experience low energy levels, but they will also experience severe issues maintaining positive relationships and overall well-being.

Energy and Mental Health

There are numerous factors that can contribute to mental health issues. As previously discussed, societal issues and unresolved grief and trauma can yield higher levels of anxiety, depression, and PTSD. It is also very common for people to suffer from mood disorders, personality disorders, disordered eating, substance abuse, etc. The list is long for psychological ailments and how they happen, and it has been proven that 1 in 3 people will be diagnosed with a mental illness in their lifetime. Even without a specific disorder, most people will have periods of life where their mental health suffers greatly.

No matter what a person's struggle with mental health looks like, or what they are doing (or not doing) in terms of treatment, the body expends a lot of energy when a part of it is unwell.

Daily Energy Regulation

No matter what it is in your life that is causing you to feel depleted, it is vital to pay attention to the energy fields within the body and identify the areas of greatest pain and imbalance. In the spectrum of health, people often take measures such as going to see the doctor, therapist, or grief counselor, taking medication, and making lifestyle changes such as finding a hobby or increasing exercise. However, a piece that is commonly overlooked in the healing journey is healing energetically. No matter how much you invest in your mental, physical, emotional, and spiritual health, if your energies remain imbalanced, it is impossible to reach a state of full wellness. That being said, energy healing is the missing piece in most people's quests for holistic health.

In many cases, it can be beneficial to seek the help of energy healers, massage therapists, and reiki, craniosacral therapy, or bodywork practitioners. These practitioners are trained in getting in touch with your energy centers and helping bring them back into balance through healing touch, body movements, and visualization techniques. If you are dealing with energy imbalance, seeing a practitioner can be an excellent investment in unlocking your highest levels of health and joy in life.

It is also possible to use a variation of the body scan mediation from chapter 3 to check in with your energy levels on your own. By taking notice of the sensations in each area of your body, you can come closer in touch with any area of your body where you experience regular pain, tension, or other unpleasant feelings. This is often a sign of imbalance or trapped energy. Additionally, the tense and release technique in each area of the body can yield healing and balance by releasing negative energy and tension. It is important to check in with yourself daily, asking your body where energy may be trapped or depleted and what you can do to replenish yourself.

Chapter 3: The Daily Energy Healing Journey

Understanding Your Energy Field: Daily Energy Healing Meditation with Journaling (Week 5)

There is a great variety when it comes to human energy fields. People experience varying levels of sensitivity to the energy of other people and the environment. Some people are incredibly in tune with "vibes"; others are empaths who feel the emotional experiences of others on a deep level, while still others experience very little of either. There is also a lot of variation in the way people recharge energetically, as well as what depletes them. In the common case of introverts and extroverts, for example, introverts need time alone to replenish their energy and feel balanced, while extroverts recharge in stimulating environments with other people around. One of the first steps to protecting your personal energetic field is to understand how it works.

Understanding Your Energy Field Journal Prompt (Week 5):

When you feel exhausted and not like yourself, which activities are most likely to replenish your energy? Do you enjoy a night out with friends? Yoga? A walk in the park? Leisure reading? Finding a new adventure? Taking a bubble bath? Listening to your favorite music on blast? List 5-10 activities that help you gain balance and feel energized.

Now, make a list of the things that make you feel most drained. These can be large things, like a specific task at your job, or small things like doing the dishes. You may find that you feel drained if you spend too much time alone or, consequently, when you spend too much time around other people.

When it comes to activities that make you feel drained, ask yourself to what extent that specific thing is necessary in your life. If you find yourself feeling drained from spending too much time around other people, for example, you can easily make a change by scheduling more "nothing time" or "alone time" into your days and taking the time you need to replenish. Household tasks and daily responsibilities are necessary, but by being aware of the ones that drain you the most, you can bring more attention to the process and doing what you need to replenish energy before or after.

Protecting Your Energy Field: Daily Energy Healing Meditation with Journaling (Week 6)

Close your eyes and ask yourself, "what does my energy field look like?" Write down any specific colors, textures, shapes, or patterns of movement.

Once you have an image in your mind of your energy field, ask yourself, "What does it look like for outside energies to enter my field?" Write down what healthy and unhealthy outside energies look like.

Then ask yourself, "How can I regulate the energies entering my field? What does it look like when I decide what I will let in?" Describe this process.

Finally, ask yourself, "How does my body feel when I regulate what I allow to enter my energy field?" Write down everything that comes to mind.

Healing Through Trapped Emotion Release: Daily Energy Healing Meditation with Journaling (Week 7)

In our society, we are often faced with life circumstances that force us to repress our basic human emotions. It is very possible for anger, rage, or grief to become stuck in the body because it is considered "impractical" to have those reactions in public. Similarly, we often hear about people being described as "annoyingly happy" or "overly emotional." Most of us are taught not only to manage our emotions but to distance ourselves from them and react emotionally only in certain contexts. Additionally, we tend to suppress negative emotions such as fear, shame, inadequacy, and insecurity, for the purpose of appearing like we have everything together. Between life events and societal expectations, it is very easy for the emotions we suppress to become trapped in our bodies, which can create adverse health effects, negatively impact our relationships, and keep us from living our best lives.

Begin by making a list of as many emotions as you can think of

Run down the list of emotions one by one, asking yourself, "Is there anywhere in my body I am holding *particular emotion*?"

Write down the emotions you feel are trapped. Take some time to journal about how certain emotions arose, or times when you felt you had to suppress your emotions.

With each emotion you have labeled as being trapped, write: "I give myself permission to release this *particular emotion*

Cultivating Self-Trust in your Healing Journey: Daily Energy Healing
Meditation With Journaling (Week 8)

No matter what you do in your life, there will always be people who don't
understand the choices you make, or who judge the path you are on. When
it comes to renewing and protecting your energy, there is no room for
anyone else's opinions or emotions in regards to your journey. It requires
a great deal of self-trust to go your own way and let what other people
think about it roll off your back. For this reason, it is vital to begin
everyday establishing a sense of self-trust with your own journey and
energy management skills. The following four journal questions will help
you direct your energy before going about your day.

What are you most grateful for today?

What are your intentions for how you will direct your energy today?

What are your fears/things you perceive as a potential threat?

What are your commitments to yourself and the world?

Mini Meditation Toolbox: 25 Quick and Easy Energy Restoration and Protection Meditations

One-Minute Energy Cleanse

- This meditation is useful if you find yourself with a person or in a specific situation that feels negative or energetically draining. You do not need to be alone to complete this meditation

- Pause where you are and allow yourself to take a few deep, cleansing breaths

- Focus exclusively on your breathing; you may close your eyes or leave them open

- Feel the inner power within the core of your body, around your abdomen. Remind yourself that you are in control and have the power to maintain balance.

- As you inhale, pull love, light, and peace into your body

- As you exhale, breathe out pain, annoyance, and toxicity

Energy from the Earth

- Begin by entering a space in nature. This can be on the beach, in the mountains, near a river, in a garden, by the lake, or in your own yard

- If possible, slip your shoes off, so your bare feet are in contact with the earth

- Start with a few cleansing breaths, taking note of everything you see, hear, smell, and feel in your environment

- Placing the soles of your feet on the ground, begin to breathe, pulling the energy from the earth up through your body

- Remember that you are One with the nature that courses around you. Allow it to heal what is broken within you and leave you feeling rejuvenated

Re-Centering Head Hold (3-5 minute meditation)

- Close your eyes and place the palm of one hand horizontally across the crown of your head, and the other palm across your forehead (over the energetic points of the Crown and Third Eye chakras). This position can be done while standing, sitting, or lying down.

- While clutching your head in this position, bring attention to any sensations in your body. What needs your attention most right now?

- Allow yourself to come back to the present moment, feeling grounded in your body and in your experience

- Breathe in awareness, focus, and comfort, exhaling anxiety and distraction

- When you open your eyes, notice how you feel grounded in your space

The Cloak of Protection

- This meditation is useful for energy protection before going out into the world, whether that is to work, the supermarket, an appointment, etc.

- Although you do not know what kinds of energies you may encounter, or which people may try to take your energy from you, remind yourself that you are in control of your own energy and that you have the capacity to protect yourself

- Close your eyes and imagine a dark-blue, almost black cloak made of a soft, thick material like a velvet night sky. The cloak is full-length with a hood to protect all of your chakras.

- Imagine a ray of light outlining the cloak in whatever color(s) feel most magical, protective, and authentic to who you are

- Set off into the world knowing that you are safe within yourself and your energy cloak and that you do not need to be afraid

De-Cluttering your Space

- When energy is lacking or out of balance, the spaces we live in are likely to reflect that imbalance with clutter and messiness. The more we feel like we "don't have our lives together," the more likely we are to have a messy desk, dishes piling up in the sink, laundry that still needs to be folded, or a car that has not been cleared of trash

- Such spaces do not allow for peace and mental clarity and can be even more draining to come back to after a long day

- Dedicate yourself to one area of your life to de-clutter. This can be your kitchen, your car, your bedroom, etc. Close your eyes before beginning and take a few deep, cleansing breaths to approach the task calmly

- Begin to address all of the clutter in the space, not only picking it up but putting it into a designated area where it can be organized and easy to find

- You may find that you want to create a special shelf or move some furniture around to make the space less cluttered. As you go, notice the energy that continues to unfold in your body

- When you finish, place a "clutter basket" in your room, the car, the living room, etc. where you can compile all the clutter throughout the day and put it away before bed

De-Cluttering your Mind (5-minute meditation)

- Close your eyes and begin to breathe deeply

- Ask yourself, "What is taking up the most space in my mind right now?"

- Bring your attention to whatever it is that is distracting you, and why it makes you feel out of control

- Breathe into that situation, saying, "I have control over this situation, and I am not going to let it spill out into the rest of my day. I am clearing this space."

The Energy-Ownership Mantra

- This meditation is ideal to perform in the morning, or before going out to interact with the world or other people

- Sit in a place where you feel energized (on the porch, in your meditation corner, etc.)

- Close your eyes and begin to breathe, checking in with any unresolved emotions or senses within the body

- Now begin to picture your energy field. Say to yourself: "My energy field is my sacred space, and other energies will only permeate it when I allow them to."

- Breathe into this thought for several moments

- Now, bring this thought into your mental space: "I have the wisdom to discern what belongs to me and what belongs to other people. I can be empathetic and attentive to other people's emotions, struggles, and opinions without assuming responsibility for them."

Epsom Bath Energy Renewal

- Begin by selecting your favorite scented Epsom salts. You may also customize your bath with petals, oils, and candles as according to the healing plants, herbs, and oils listed in Chapter 4

- Run a hot bath, letting your Epsom salts and other elements saturate the water

- Customize your space with the light of candles, meditative music, and anything else that makes you feel at peace

- Find a comfortable position inside the tub. Close your eyes, and feel your entire body relax into the heat and gentle movement of the water.

- Begin to conduct a body scan, feeling entirely vulnerable to this moment at peace with only yourself

- Ask your body, "What do I need right now?"

- The water should be hot enough that you begin to sweat (be sure to have a glass of water nearby). As you sweat, imagine your body purging itself of every blockage, every impurity, and every negativity

Sealing your Energy Field

- Close your eyes and begin to breathe

- Bring the image of your energy field to your mind. You may picture a wall, a bubble, or a glowing ring of light (this image may also differ depending on the day)

- Picture what other energies look like, floating around your field like particles in an atom. Say to yourself, "I am in control of what comes in."

- Imagine yourself recognizing people who are trying to take your energy or bear their burdens. Imagine any fear, anger, or resentment you may feel.

- Say to yourself, "No, not today." Imagine your bubble becoming impermeable, your wall being sealed, your glowing ring of light rejecting anything that does not belong inside

- Allow yourself to feel empowered over your energy, without feeling any resentment or judgment towards those who once posed a threat

Building your Sanctuary

- Sit down and close your eyes, beginning to breathe into yourself

- With each breath, ask yourself, "What makes me feel safe?" Repeat three times.

- Switch the phrase to "What makes me feel at peace?" Repeat three times.

- Switch the phrase to "What makes me feel loving?" Repeat three times

- Switch to "What makes me feel joy?"

- Lastly, ask yourself, "What makes me feel renewed?"

- When you ask yourself these questions, you may see certain crystals, scenes in nature, types of music, plants, aromas, decorations, activities, or color schemes. Take note of whatever comes to mind.

- Use these things that come to you in meditation to mindfully cultivate a space for yourself to come into every day when you need time to recharge. This can be a meditation corner, a spot in the backyard, or any other space that is sacred to you and provides feelings of security and rest.

Cultivating Non-Reaction

- This meditation can be used when encountering a stressful situation, having a difficult conversation, or otherwise entering a state of nervous or angry energy

- Before responding to whatever the negative stimulant is, breathe into the moment. Close your eyes if needed.

- Tell yourself, "I can choose not to expend energy on this interaction. I can choose to move peacefully into the next moment."

- Feel the tension within you melt away as you make the choice not to internalize the stress of the situation or the negative energy coming at you

Boundary Setting

- Find a quiet place to sit and self-reflect. Breathe into the moment

- After you have settled into your breath, ask yourself, "What people, circumstances, or tasks drain my energy and leave me feeling agitated or exhausted?"

- Allow the answers to rise into your consciousness at will. Meditate on every name, every task, every circumstance which makes you feel tense and throws your energy out of balance.

- With each name, circumstance, and task, say to yourself, "This *person, place, thing* has no power over me. I can maintain my energy in spite of it."

- Next, ask yourself, "Where do I need to draw the line with this *person, place, thing*?"

- Listen to your intuition tell you what your boundaries should be. Perhaps, this looks like gently cutting off a toxic person, or limiting your interaction time with them. It could be quitting a job that is no longer good for you or asking for accommodations to make your environment more positive. It could be telling someone who expects you to bear their burdens that their energies are no longer your responsibility. Or, perhaps it is to establish a self-care activity to do directly after a draining task.

Trigger Awareness

- If your energy has ever been thrown out of balance by trauma, there are likely still factors of your environment that can strike at any time, causing your body to react in the same way it did at the time of the trauma.

- Breathe into the moment, asking yourself, "what elements of my environment cause me to lose control of my logic and feel afraid, helpless, irrational, in pain, or otherwise unbalanced or unhealthy energetically."

- These elements are called "triggers." Bring your awareness to these triggers, simply allowing them to be there without judgment.

- Say to yourself, "that moment in time is over. I can now release myself."

Energetic Tapping

- Begin by determining 3-5 affirmations or manifestations for the day ahead ("I manifest peace," "I am content," "I am present," "I manifest energy," "I am growing," "I manifest healing," "I manifest loving-kindness," etc.)
- Breathe deeply, pondering the affirmations/manifestations
- Choose your first manifestation/affirmation. With your index and middle fingers on both hands, begin tapping lightly on the crown of your head, repeating the manifestation or affirmation three times
- Move to the temples, tapping and saying the manifestation/affirmation three times
- Repeat at the inner corners of the brow bone
- Repeat just above the brow line
- Repeat at the top of the cheekbones
- Repeat below the ear lobes at the crest of the jawbone
- Repeat at the top of the chest
- Repeat on the left wrist, then switch to the right wrist
- Switch to the next affirmation/manifestation and go through the process again, staying in touch with your breath throughout

Listening to your Intuition

- Find a space where you feel completely comfortable and relaxed
- Begin to breathe deeply, coming into the present moment
- Ask yourself, "What does my inner self need me to know right now?"
- Keep breathing, holding space for whatever answer arises
- If necessary, you can ask follow-up questions to yourself, like "Is there any threat I need to be prepared to protect myself from?" or "How can I best love the world today?" Or "What do I need to do to take care of myself today?"
- Continue to breathe and hold space, trusting that your heart will guide you to make the correct decisions for yourself

Memory Reclamation (specifically for healing of trauma victims)

- Find a space where you feel totally safe and undisturbed. It is best to do this meditation on a day where you can invest in self-care and rest.
- Begin to breathe, telling yourself, "I am safe. I am safe. I am safe."
- Allow the memory of a particularly traumatic event to come to your mind. Continue to breathe, telling yourself, "I am safe."

- Pay attention to the details of that memory. What do you see? What do you hear? What do you feel?

- As the memory progresses, allow it to release its energetic hold on your body. Tell yourself, "That was then. This is now. I am safe."

- Feel the trauma release its hold on you, restoring itself to a basic memory of the past

Defining your Needs

- Sit in a peaceful place, breathing into the moment

- Bring attention to any pain or unrest within your body. Without judgment, allow it to be there, asking if there is anything you should learn from it.

- Generally, where there is pain or unrest, there is a need being left unmet. Ask yourself, "What is it that I need?"

- Allow your needs to arise into your consciousness ("I need a day off for my mental health," "I need a trip into nature," "I need a bath," "I need a warm, nourishing meal," "I need to go to sleep early," etc.)

- Breathe into each need, envisioning yourself meeting that particular need

- Ask yourself, "Is there anyone else I need to make aware of these needs?"

- Envision yourself having a calm conversation about your needs with your boss, your partner, your family, or a friend. Envision them, reacting gently and yourself feeling better understood and supported.

- Continue to breathe into your capacity to meet your energetic needs and make those needs known to others.

"Nothing Time"

- Set aside a minimum of one hour of time with absolutely nothing scheduled

- Sit down, breathing into the moment. Tell yourself, "this is my time. I have nowhere to be, nothing to do; I do not need to feel rushed."

- Allow your deepest intuition to guide your next step. Do whatever comes to mind first

- While you proceed with your "nothing time," allow your breath to guide every move

Discovering your Support System

- Bring your attention to the present moment, focusing on your breath

- Ask yourself, "Who of the people I know understands and embraces me for who I truly am?"

- Breathe with each name that comes up, allowing loving-kindness and appreciation for that person to flow through your body

- Ask yourself, "Who in my life encourages me to reach my full potential?

- Repeat the action of breathing with each name that arises

- Ask yourself, "Who in my life do I feel most at rest with?"

- Repeat the action of breathing with each name that arises

- Continue to breathe, saying to yourself, "These are my people. This is my support system. I will allow myself to lean on them when I need to."

Glowing Love-Energy

- Find a restful position and begin to breathe

- Imagine the aura of your energy field. How big is it? What color is it?

- Say to yourself, "I am pure love. I have room to love the entire universe and everything in it."

- Continue to repeat this phrase with every breath. Picture the aura expanding and glowing brighter

Jaguar Spirit Animal Protection

- Bring yourself into the present moment with deep breathing

- From the depth of your being, say, "I call on the spirit of the jaguar to protect me."

- Feel the reverberations of the jaguar's protection through your body, aiding you in repelling negative energy and toxicity
- Imagine a fierce, beautiful guard of your energy field, encircling you with fierce love and security

Energetic Breathing (1-3-minute meditation)

- Take some space away from your everyday life (in the bathroom, in the car, etc.) to just breathe
- Implement the 5-5-7 breathing technique
- With every breath in, say to yourself, "I breathe in pure energy."
- With every breath out, say to yourself, "I breathe out *exhaustion, *toxicity, *negativity, etc."
- Continue until you feel the tingle of pure energy coursing through your veins

Energetic Dancing/Movement

- Find a space where you can be alone and feel completely secure
- Play a song that stirs your soul and emotions, causing you to have a visceral reaction in the body each time you hear it
- As the song begins, close your eyes and deep breathe, maybe swaying back and forth slightly

- When you feel ready, release your body to move as it feels led. No choreography, no expectations, simply letting the movement of the moment lead your body into a state of pure surrender and release

- Surrender entirely to the moment, trusting your body to release any tension or trauma

- Give your body the space and freedom to heal, coming into energetic harmony

The Art of Saying "No"

- Close your eyes and begin to breathe deeply

- Begin to consider the things that drain your energy. Perhaps you have a tendency to overcommit or find yourself stuck in a relationship or circumstance that no longer serves you. Breathe with each of these places where you feel stuck

- Say to yourself "I have the power to say 'no.'"

- Imagine yourself having the necessary conversation, turning down the opportunity, or simply choosing to remove yourself from the situation

- Feel the power of saying no and being in full control of where you place your energy

The Restorative Power of Letting Go

- Breathe deeply, cultivating a sense of full peace and security

- Ask yourself, "Where are the parts of me that I need to get back?"

- Take notice of every person or place that comes to mind as still having a part of your energy and your essence

- If there are any feelings of melancholy, nostalgia, resentment, shame, or anger, allow them to be there, breathing as they flow through you

- Say to yourself, "I release this *person or place*. I reclaim what they have that is rightfully mine."

- Continue to breathe into this empowerment

PART V

Finding Your Way Back to the Present Moment

Chapter 1: Back to the Basics

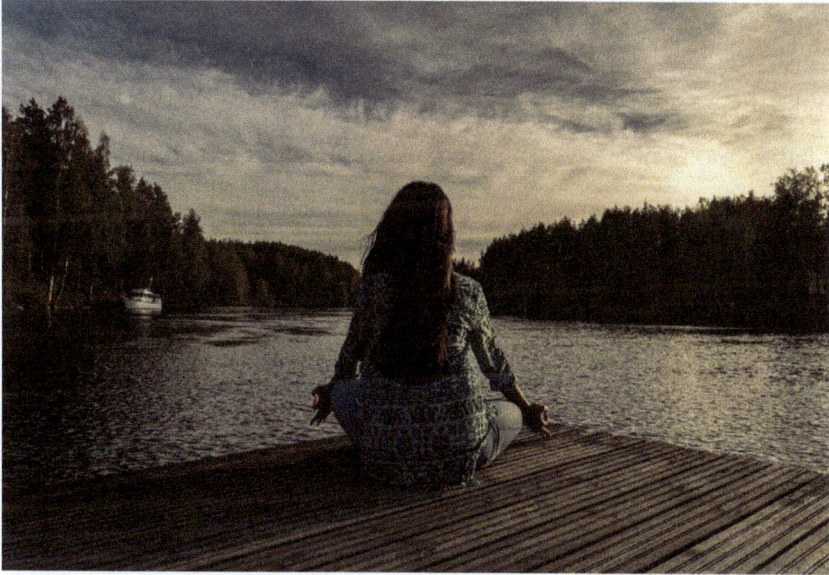

When most people think of mindfulness, they envision monks or yogis, sitting cross legged for hours with closed eyes and poised fingers overlooking the Himalayas. Although mindfulness is present in the lives of monks and yogis, what most people don't know is how easy it is to incorporate mindfulness into our everyday lives. As a matter of fact, a mindful state is the most natural and restful state for human beings—a state in which we were all living and moving in as children. If you think back to your childhood, you will likely remember that your concept of time and perception of reality was much different. Most children are very in touch with their emotions, letting them come and go naturally. If a child falls down in one moment and skins their knee, the child will likely begin to cry. However, if a few moments later they are being offered ice cream, their tears will dry, and they will continue on with their day. Mindfulness is the reason children are so in tune with the details of life that adults seem to miss. It is also the reason they are more likely to screech with joy, run around excitedly in enjoyable environments, wake up easily in the morning, and take the time they need to calm down from anger or sadness until the next happy moment arises. Children spend very little time thinking about things beyond the present moment. Even if they have something to look forward to, they are still likely to become invested in the moment at hand, whether that is playing, enjoying time with their parents, or eating a meal. So, what happens as people grow older that brings us away from this natural state of mindfulness?

There are a number of factors that pull people out of the present moment. From the time a child begins elementary school, they are presented with a schedule for the day, which remains relatively the same. Children are expected to remain within the structures presented to them, and the idea of forward-thinking and preparing for the next hour's activity becomes introduced. As they grow, children will likely have more expectations placed upon them, whether those expectations are academic, extracurricular, or within the home. Of course, it is necessary for children to learn how to be responsible and dedicate the time they need to the important things in life. However, as they become further exposed to the constant rush and future-oriented thinking of their parents and teachers, they come to see time as something that no longer belongs to them to fully inhabit.

Furthermore, as people approach teenage and young adulthood, they will begin to face challenges that most children are either shielded from or otherwise unaware of. People become flooded with the pressure to perform well and always be doing more today than yesterday. Although the expectations of cultures and societies vary, we can be sure that people are overwhelmed with the pressure to meet those expectations in order to be considered successful and valid. Once one bar is crossed, another one is waiting, and there is no time to slack. Additionally, the older people become, the more likely they are to be subject to long-lasting pain in their lives. This can come in the form of relationships ending, failing to accomplish something, being mistreated by other people, losing and grieving loved ones, or coming to terms with painful childhood events that did not make sense at the time. Teenagers become increasingly subject to mental health issues as they advance into adulthood, having to face all of the hard realities of the world and still come out on top. People may also be subject to trauma as a result of illness, accident, or abuse. All of these factors are enough to work against people and pull them out of the present moment, either because it is too painful to be there, or because they are simply too distracted.

Human beings experience over 60,000 thoughts per day, but the vast majority are dedicated either to planning for the future or worrying about the past. Becoming overly concerned about the future or steeping in the pains or regrets of the past can increase levels of stress in the body, which makes people more anxious and prone to physical health problems.

The mind naturally wanders, and it is impossible to keep thoughts from coming. Mindfulness is not a tool to eradicate such thoughts, as is the common misconception. Rather, it is a tool through which to acknowledge the thoughts the mind creates, bring attention to them, and allow them to move through. This ultimately brings people into what is happening here and now and gives them more control over their minds and how they orient themselves in their environments.

Because mindfulness is a skill that all human beings are equipped with at our core, it is something that can be re-learned. Just as we exercise our bodies to strengthen our muscles, so we must work to strengthen our brain through mindfulness. The way this strengthening happens is through being aware of thoughts as they arise, then breathing back into the present moment. The more practice is given to returning to the present moment, the stronger the mind will become in remaining in the present more often. Just as the body physically strengthens and becomes healthier over time with exercise, mindfulness exercises can physically change the structure of the brain to make it healthier. Mindfulness activates the positive components of the hippocampus, which is the part of the brain responsible for good things like creativity, joy, and the ability to process emotions. This, in turn, decreases stress levels, depressive tendencies, addictive behaviors, and the fight or flight instinct by shrinking the part of the brain responsible for negative things (the amygdala). Overall, increased mindfulness is the key to a longer, healthier, more creative, and more joyful life.

Chapter 2: Unlocking Your True Purpose Through Mindfulness

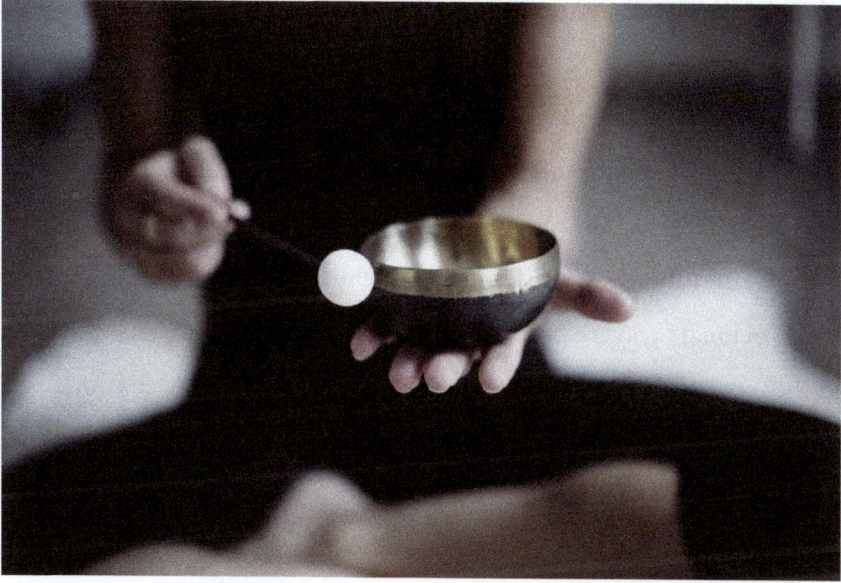

Re-centering Yourself

Everyone has days where everything seems to be spinning out of control, and there seems to be no way to manage the chaos. The days where you wake up late, run late to work, spill coffee on your shirt, get cut off on the road, get yelled at by your boss, spend the entire day at work in a confused frenzy, only to come home and bicker with your partner. Since the beginning of time, the human mind has been conditioned to release stress hormones and illicit the fight or flight instinct for the purpose of protection and survival. In the past, this primal instinct was very useful for escaping threats. As times have changed, the threats have become less severe, but the brain's response has remained largely the same. Now, these fight or flight reactions are likely to be triggered by everyday scenarios, such as those previously detailed. The hormone-induced responses that occur when we're stressed out are quick to send us spiraling into emotionally dramatic, and far less peaceful dimensions.

The good news is, mindfulness can be used as a tool for re-centering and gaining control over your anxiety and emotional reactions when you start to feel yourself spiral. Although there is no way to avoid stress and drama in daily life, mindfulness can serve as a shield of calm presence to protect your well-being. If you are preparing to enter a situation that you anticipate could be stressful, like a high-stakes day at work, a scary doctor's appointment, or a difficult conversation with a loved one, it can be incredibly helpful to bring yourself down to a more calm and balanced state in preparation for the stress you are about to deal with. You may find yourself with a racing heart, sweating palms, an unclear head, and the feeling of "butterflies in your stomach." Another area where it is common to feel these physical effects of anxiety is when encountering dramatic situations. Drama can arise tense moments with other people, as well as within the theoretical situations people create for themselves when worrying about what they cannot control (for example, the perception other people have of them, or events that may or may not occur in the future). Giving attention to what is happening in your mind and body and allowing yourself to breathe into the moment can be a total lifesaver in moments of drama or stress. Two to three minutes of deep breathing in your car before going to work, or taking a few deep breaths before reacting in a tense moment, can make a drastic difference in your sense of balance and your ability to deal with stress without launching into fight or flight.

Giving Your Emotions Space

The goal of mindfulness is not to eliminate emotions, but rather, to gain control over the impact they have on how we orient ourselves in the world. It is vital to honor our emotions and give them space to exist and teach us, without letting them seize control. Mindfulness is an excellent tool for giving our emotions space in this way. When an emotion arises, mindfulness gives us a chance to observe that emotion without judgment. In this calm space, we can ask our emotions, "What are you trying to teach me?" We can more clearly discern why we are experiencing a certain emotion, and become in touch with the deeper needs that may have caused that emotion to arise. Just as a child may cry when they need to be nourished our held, we may find ourselves growing angry or agitated when we need support, touch, or self-care. Similarly, we may find ourselves feeling stressed or anxious in scenarios that are subconsciously triggering moments from the past. In these cases, our stress and anxiety are begging us to become in touch with our past self, reminding ourselves that we are safe, and the traumatic moments from the past are over. Once our emotions have been given a non-judgmental space to exist, they can smoothly and peacefully move through the body and be released. This frees us to move from moment to moment like children do, without being constrained by unresolved emotions. Additionally, giving this space to our emotions in mindfulness helps to temper our reactions, which can prevent us from acting out in extreme ways and potentially doing or saying something we regret.

Making Clear Decisions

With the human mind constantly being muddled with thoughts, it can be hard to see things clearly. Sometimes our minds are cluttered by the expectations flying at us from every different direction, or perhaps by our fears of what will happen if things don't go to plan. When it comes to making decisions, we are often faced with numerous options, and it can be difficult to navigate through the chaos in our minds to come to a well thought out resolution. In a distracted, anxious, or removed state, our minds are like a pond on a rainy day—rippling to a point where there is no more clarity. Mindfulness is the calming of the waters, which brings us to a place where we can more clearly think of all possible outcomes of a decision and check in with what we truly need before moving into the next moment.

Keeping Yourself Safe

Although fight or flight instincts originally developed as a way to keep humans safe, in many modern-day scenarios, they do quite the opposite. Let's go back to the example from the beginning of the chapter about the chain of events in a typical chaotic day. If you wake up late in the morning and rush to make your coffee, not paying attention to what you are doing, you run the risk of haphazardly screwing the lid on your to-go cup, then sloshing boiling hot coffee over the edge of the cup and onto yourself as you bolt out the door. Although such a scenario could simply result in a stained shirt, the inattentiveness could have a more drastic effect, such as burning yourself or someone else. Driving to work in a state of panic over running late causes you to be more likely to break the rules of the road— driving too fast, making dangerous decisions when changing lanes, taking turns too fast, running yellow lights just before they turn red, etc. Additionally, the panicked state can lead to anger with yourself or others on the road, which can further impair judgment and put you at greater risk of an accident. Attempting to have a conversation with your boss if you are in fight or flight mode could result in being overly emotional and saying or doing something extreme which could place you at odds within your workplace, potentially even costing your position. Going throughout your day in a frenzy causes you to be less aware of what is going on around you, which can lead to further threats to safety like leaving a burner on, forgetting to eat or drink enough water, or neglecting those in your care (such as pets or children) as a result of your own inner distractions. Finally, as stress from the day carries into the home at the end of the day, it can pose a major threat to relationships. The more stressed out and less clear thinking you are, the more likely you are to say or do something threatening to your partner, to put yourself in an aggressive and volatile situation, and to make brash decisions that have the potential to haunt your future.

Improving Relationships

Just as we must give ourselves space to learn, grow, and process our experiences, we must give that space to those around us as well. When a partner or friend is acting in a way we don't enjoy, mindfulness can allow us to take a step back and look at the situation from a position of empathy. We can allow ourselves to hold space for whatever that person may be going through individually and express our support while also maintaining boundaries and staying in control of what we can. Everyone is deserving of space to be listened to, understood, and supported for who they are. However, it is incredibly difficult to give that space to anyone if it has not been cleared within oneself.

When we operate out of a mindless state, there is hardly any space to meet our own needs and process our own experience, much less to provide that to other people. This can lead us to be closed off to the ones we love, push them away, or act out in anger, selfishness, or aggression. If we have not given space to what is going on within us, we cannot offer full empathy to others. Only 20% of the population is recorded to practice true empathy, which can be linked to the rarity of true mindfulness among adults. Mindfulness allows us to be more present to our own needs in order to hold adequate space for the needs of others as well.

Attention and mutual respect are core elements of every functional relationship. Practicing mindfulness can improve relationships with all the people in our lives by preparing us for every engagement and calming our minds enough to be fully present in the moments we share with others. Mindfulness clears the space for us to listen intentionally to other people and pay more attention to what kind of people they are and what kind of support they need. It allows us to love other people better by increasing our awareness of how they feel most loved. By being present in the moment at hand, as opposed to trapped in the past or future, you are more likely to remember to pick up the phone and give your grandmother a call, to be fully engaged when interacting with your child, or to remember the kind of kombucha your significant other likes best from the store. Not only does mindfulness allow for more meaningful conversations and joyful memories, but it also increases the functionality of our relationships overall so that both ourselves and those we love are feeling fully respected, listened to, and encouraged.

Fostering True Joy

We often hear the term "childlike joy" to describe moments of pure bliss, enthusiasm, and full satisfaction. As people grow into adults, such moments tend to be few and far between, with many remembering the most joyful moments to have been those that occurred in childhood. The expectations of daily life become too much, and most people find themselves trapped in a cycle of constant anticipation. People spend so much time thinking about where they would rather be (on vacation, in bed, enjoying the weekend) that the days melt into each other without us realizing all the moments of our lives we are missing. The biggest societal misconception is that true happiness lies in what we do not yet have. We are flooded with lies such as "Once I can buy this new TV, then I'll be happy," or, "Once I have a partner, then I'll be happy," or, "I'll be happy once I can say I've been to five different countries." Mindfulness abolishes these lies by proving to us that the capacity for true joy lies not in the future but in the here and now. Wherever you are right now, whatever you have, and whichever stage of life you're in, mindfulness reminds you that *this* is your chance to experience beauty and satisfaction like never before. Take time to look at the flowers you did not notice growing in front of your neighbor's house, the complexity of coffee's flavor as it slides down your throat, the way your loved one's eyes crinkle when they smile, the laughter of a child, every intricate flavor of dinner, or the unique people wandering up and down the streets you drive every day to work. It is here that joy resides; all you have to do is be present enough to recognize it.

Chapter 3: Moving Mindfully in Daily Life

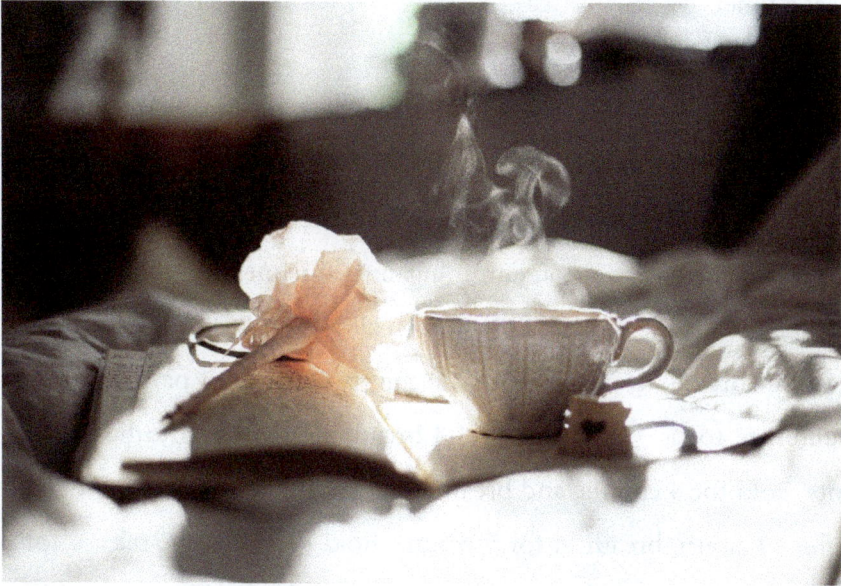

Coming to the Present Moment: Daily Guided Mindfulness Meditation With Journaling (Week 1)

Cultivating Mindfulness

This meditation should be done in a space where you feel fully comfortable, safe, and relaxed. Perhaps it is in a corner of your bedroom, in a garden, by your favorite lake, or even in your car. Make sure you can fully relax and avoid distractions. Some people meditate best with instrumental music or nature sounds in the background, while others prefer silence. Feel free to try multiple methods and see which is most soothing to you (this can vary depending on the day). You may do this meditation sitting in a chair, on a mat, or lying flat on your back with your palms up to the sky. You will need to give yourself 5-20 minutes of time to practice, depending on your skill level and current state. If you like, you can set a timer.

Start by coming into the moment with a few deep breaths. Settle into your body and take note of any sensations you feel. If you feel pain, tingling, warmth, or tightness in any part of your body, focus your breath into that space. Imagine any tension unfurling into openness. Notice as your thoughts arise. Take notice of them, then allow them to pass as you come back to the breath. If it is helpful, you can try a breathing pattern in order to culminate focus. To do the 4-4-4 breathing pattern, breathe in for 4 counts, hold for 4 counts, and breathe out for 4 counts. To do the 5-5-7 breathing pattern, breath in for 5 counts, hold for 5 counts, release for 7 counts. Sometimes it helps to imagine breathing in the things you wish to see more of in your daily life (creativity, love, patience, openness) and exhale the negative things (fear, negativity, sadness, stress). Allow yourself to spend a few moments in a more active state of breathing in, releasing, and paying attention to your body.

With practice, you may enter a state where your thoughts slow and you become fully grounded in the present moment. In this state, you are no longer bombarded with thoughts, nor distracted by elements of your environment. It becomes easier to return to the breath. All restlessness and tension in the body seem to melt away, and the mind reaches a flowing, liquified state. There may be days when you cannot enter into this state, and you remain restless throughout the course of the meditation. If this happens, allow it to be that way, observing every thought that arises, then letting it go.

After the time is up, begin to arrive in the moment by moving your body slightly—wiggling your fingers and toes, tensing and releasing your muscles, etc. Next, you're your eyes. Notice how bright and clear the world looks to mindful eyes. Notice the calm, transcendent feeling in your body, and continue to move with it as you go about your day.

Mindfulness Meditation Journal Prompt (Week 1):

What did you feel in your body before beginning? What do you feel now?

Which thoughts continued to arise in your consciousness? Could these thoughts have been trying to teach you something or speak to a deeper need you may have?

How does the world look after opening your eyes? What do you notice?

Come back after going about your day for several hours. Did you bring mindfulness with you into the world? If so, how?

Coming to the Present Moment: Daily Guided Mindfulness Meditation With Journaling (Week 2)

Taking Mindfulness Into the World

This meditation will be done with your eyes open in moments if your daily life. This is not a specific meditation you have to set aside time for, but rather a state you come into. Notice where your attention goes in a given moment. If your attention is drawn to a particular sight, like the nearest tree or a view from the top of a mountain, allow yourself to see it fully. Repeatedly tell yourself, "see, see, see." Breathe as you allow your eyes to truly become totally focused and take in the image fully, allowing it to become a part of your awareness.

If your attention is drawn to an auditory experience, such as the sound of cars on a city street, a rushing body of water, or an internal monologue, give full attention to that thing. Soak in that auditory experience, breathing slowly and telling yourself, "hear, hear, hear."

You may also be drawn to a particular physical or emotional experience within the body. This experience may be positive, like a pleasant bodily sensation or a feeling of joy. It may also be negative, like physical pain, or feelings of anger or feel. Either way, allow yourself to become fully present with what is there, breathing into the experience and seeing what it has to teach you. Breathe into that bodily experience, telling yourself, "feel, feel, feel."

Throughout the day, you'll find that your attention is pulled in various directions. Mindfulness is the choice to tune in to whichever place you're going in a given moment and give full attention to that experience for whatever it is.

Mindfulness Meditation Journal Prompt (Week 2):

How difficult was it to bring mindfulness into your daily life in this way? Where did you face the most challenges?

Did your attention tend towards certain experiences (visual, auditory, bodily) more than others?

Describe a specific moment where you brought mindfulness to your experience and felt truly present. What did you observe?

Coming to the Present Moment: Daily Guided Mindfulness Meditation With Journaling (Week 3)

Mindfulness at Work (or School)

The first part of this meditation should happen in a place outside of work, where you feel safe, calm, and separated from the issues you may face in the workplace. Start by identifying your biggest struggles at work. The journal portion will give you a space to write them down. Do you struggle with productivity? Boredom? Stress? Conflict resolution? Work relationships? Once you have identified your most significant area(s) of struggle, close your eyes and visualize what that unpleasant experience looks like. Perhaps it looks like you, rushing around mindlessly like a bee in a hive, stressed out and too overbooked to step away and breathe because there are more calls to make, more e-mails to send, more things to do. Or, perhaps it is the co-worker, professor, or boss that makes your stomach drop whenever you think about having to interact with them. Perhaps you feel unfulfilled at work and find yourself constantly checking the clock, thinking about the moment you get to leave. Maybe you have so many things to do and no idea where to start, so you waste a lot of time on mindless tasks. Whatever your struggles at work are, use your time and space away from work to safely visualize the situation. Breathe into the mental circumstance.

As you breathe, begin to envision what this experience would look like if it went the way you want it to. Perhaps it looks like the mental clarity that allows you to know exactly what needs to get done and how to make the best possible use of your time. It could be a greater sense of calm and courage when talking with your difficult boss or co-worker and having your message be well-received on their end. It may also be a deeper sense of satisfaction and enjoyment in the work you're doing, providing you the ability to step back and feel a sense of joy with where you're at, without constantly thinking about the next thing. Reframe the moment in your mind until you've created a mental space that feels good. Let yourself sit there, breathing, soaking it in for several minutes.

Once you go into the workplace (or school), you can bring this meditation into your life by going back to the peaceful mental image you've created over and over again. When you begin to feel stressed, bored, anxious, or unproductive, return to the space where you do not feel those things. Bring that energy into your daily work life, and watch how it revolutionizes your experience.

Mindfulness Meditation Journal Prompt (Week 3):

What do you identify as your biggest challenge(s) at work or school?

How does it look when you reframe your struggles to create a positive mental image?

What do you observe about bringing this positive mental image into difficult situations in the workplace or at school?

Mini Meditation Toolbox: 15 Quick and Easy Meditations to Integrate Mindfulness Into Your Daily Life

One-Minute Mindfulness

- Find a space where you can be alone, like on your bathroom break or in your car right before going into work, school, or home at the end of the day.
- Set a timer for one minute
- Close your eyes and focus exclusively on your breathing
- Take notice of the stresses, thoughts, and anxieties that arise, then let them go
- When you open your eyes, notice how you feel de-stressed, clear-minded, and prepared to go about your upcoming tasks and interactions with others

5-Minute Body Scan

- Set a timer for 5 minutes (if needed)
- Close your eyes and take several deep, cleansing breaths. You may use the 4-4-4 or 5-5-7 breathing patterns to deepen the breath
- Begin to bring attention to your body
- Take notice of any sensations that arise-- warmth, tingling, tension, etc.
- Bring your attention to the soles of the feet. Tighten your muscles by curling your toes, then release. What sensations do you feel?

- Continue moving up the body to your calves, hips, abdomen, chest, hands, arms, face, and neck. Observe any sensations that arise, and breathe into those sensations.

- Tighten and release the muscles in each of these areas, allowing any pent-up energy or resistance to be released

- Feel your body become grounded, relaxing completely into the floor, bed, or chair as you come into the present moment in your body and all tension melts away

Mindful Bath/Shower (10-minute meditation)

- As you begin your bath or shower, take a moment to breathe. Remove yourself from the stresses of the day and allow yourself to re-center

- Bring attention to each part of your body as you wash it

- Take notice of any sensations you feel as you move from the soles of your feet to the ends of your hair

- Breathe in the pleasant scent of the soaps and the warmth of the water. Allow yourself to feel clean, warm, and safe.

- As you wash each part of your body, thank it for what it does for you. Then, thank yourself for taking care of your body.

Mindful Morning Routine (15-30 minutes)

- Before getting out of bed, begin to stretch gently, letting thoughts come and go as your mind and body wake up. Do not rush yourself.

- Once you are ready to get out of bed, bring your attention to the space around you and the day ahead. Feel yourself become fully present in that space and prepared to move mindfully through your day

- Pay attention to every move you make, from putting on clothes, to washing your face, to setting the water on the stove to boil.

- Cultivate your awareness for the day ahead by moving slowly and calmly, one task at a time, becoming fully awake to the world

Mindful Housekeeping

- Allow yourself to become focused on the task at hand and only that task. Let every other thing you have to do or think about fade into the background.

- Bring your attention to the breath and the specific way your body moves as you complete a particular task or chore

- Give space to any thoughts or emotions that arise in your consciousness, allowing yourself to process them in a mindful state

Mindful Sit-and-Drink (10-minute meditation)

- Find a calm, quiet space where you can sit and observe the world around you (preferably outside or near a window looking outside)

- Pour a glass of your favorite tea, coffee, or cocktail to enjoy

- Eliminate all distractions. Draw your attention to the intricate flavors of the drink, and the pleasure of pulling something you enjoy into your body

- Take notice of the things happening around you. Find the things in the environment that bring you the most peace, and allow their presence with you to help you calm your mind. Become completely indulged in the moment.

Mindful Scheduling (10-minute meditation)

- Sit down with a pen and paper and center yourself with five deep breaths.

- Think about the days to come. Consider your priorities, remembering that every task is significant and an opportunity for increased mindfulness

- Ask yourself, "Am I giving myself adequate time to bring mindfulness and intentionality into each of these activities?"

- Take notice of any activities you feel you won't be able to be fully present for. Consider taking a thing or two off the list and saving them for a better time.

- Take notice of any feelings of stress, nervousness, or rush you feel in regards to your schedule. Breathe into those feelings.

- As you continue to write your schedule, allow yourself to feel empowered, in control, and prepared to be mindful of everything you are about to do

Mindful Driving

- Leave the house with plenty of time to be relaxed and focused. After entering the car, take a few moments to breathe and center yourself
- Once you start to drive, begin to take note of the things passing by. What do you see today that you did not see yesterday?
- Breathe in your visual surroundings, using them to center and remind yourself: "I am here. I am in this community. This is my life, and I am awake to it."

Mindful Walking (10-20-minute meditation)

- Choose an area where you can relax and bring attention to your surroundings. This can be in a park, in the city, on the beach, in your neighborhood, etc.
- Set out on your walk with no distractions
- Take notice of the things your eyes fall upon. If something specific catches your attention, allow yourself to pause and breathe it in.
- Pay attention to the sounds that surround you, giving yourself space to truly hear them

- Pay attention to the feeling of your feet on the pavement, the swing of your arms at your sides, and the rhythm of your breath

- Let your heart expand in curiosity and openness to whatever is ready to meet you in this space

- Allow yourself to become totally saturated with your surroundings, remembering that everything you see, hear, and feel is a part of you

Mindful Cooking and Eating

- As you enter the kitchen to prepare food, take a moment to center yourself in the moment with a few deep breaths

- Give every moment of the cooking process your full attention, from washing, to cutting, to cooking. Become fully immersed in the process (you can do this even with simple meals, like mindfully spreading peanut butter on bread)

- Breathe loving-kindness into the cooking process, remembering that the food you make will provide nourishment to yourself and others

- Once the food is ready, clear the eating space of distractions. Avoid multi-tasking

- Chew every bite of food 20-30 times, letting yourself be engulfed in the flavor and practicing gratitude for the nourishment

- Walk away from your meal feeling truly nourished and renewed

Mindful Waiting

- The next time you're trying to distract yourself at the doctor's office, the mechanic, or waiting for a friend or colleague to arrive, remind yourself that waiting is one of the most sacred times to engage in mindfulness

- Breathe into the moment, becoming aware of what surrounds you

- Bring awareness to your body. How are you feeling? Take note of any sensations

- Become aware of the thoughts that come once you stop numbing yourself with distractions. What things are running through your mind?

- Pay attention to the deeper thoughts you may have previously been ignoring. Ask yourself what you can learn about yourself and your life, or if there are any actions you need to take.

Mindful Creativity (at least 5 minutes)

- Set aside anywhere from five minutes to several hours of undivided time

- Engage in a creative project like art, writing, dancing, etc.

- Bring full presence to the creative project and try to eliminate all expectations. Allow the moment to carry you.

- Pay attention to how your mind and body react as the moment carries you. How do you feel?

- Examine what you create as a result of this free-flowing creativity

Mindful Play

- Dedicate time each week to doing something truly fun—something that makes you feel like a kid again (climbing a tree, swimming in the lake, drawing with chalk, baking cookies, having a game night, etc.)

- Eliminate all distractions and allow this to be a moment to step away from your everyday life and responsibilities

- Allow yourself to become lost in the childlike joy of play. Laugh loudly, let your body dance, be curious.

- Let the feeling of childlike joy saturate your body and carry this joy with you as you move back into your daily life.

Mindful Movement (10-30 minutes)

- Choose one of your favorite forms of movement (swimming, walking, dancing, going to the gym, etc.) and dedicate at least ten minutes to it

- As you begin to move, establish a deeper sense of body awareness. Pay attention to the feelings in your body as you begin to warm up and exercise

- Pay attention to the way your heart beats, your lungs heave, your face begins to sweat, and your body tingles with the sense of being alive

- Thank your body for all it does for you.

Mindful Listening/Quality Time

- Apply this meditation to any quality time you spend with another person, whether that is grabbing coffee or going for a walk with a loved one, interacting with co-workers, are conversing with the grocery store cashier

- Before interacting with others, bring attention to your levels of empathy. Set the intention to hold space for other people and the moments you share with them

- Eliminate distractions (like technology) and allow yourself to put everything else going on in your life on pause in order to be fully present

- One of the best ways to show love for people and to cultivate personal mindfulness is through mindful listening. Focus all of your attention on the other person and what they are saying. When you ask how their day is going, be present to hear the answer.

- Do not think of what your next move will be, what you will say, or where you will go. Simply be there, showing loving-kindness, holding space, and taking it all in.

Mini Meditation Toolbox: 10 Quick and Easy Meditations to Ease Stress, Depression, Addiction, Anxiety, Pain, Distraction, and Loss Using Mindfulness

Journaling the Consciousness (10-minute meditation)

- Sit down with a journal and a pen and set your timer for 10 minutes

- As thoughts, worries, or emotions arise, immediately write them down. Do not worry about structure, grammar, or content, just write.

- When the time is up, look over what you wrote

- Ask yourself which themes seem to reoccur. Where are you feeling stress in your life? What is occupying most of your mental space?

- Close your eyes and take a few moments to breathe and meditate on the thing(s) that need your attention the most

- Open your eyes. Notice how you feel lighter and in touch with your experience

Distraction Cleanse: Clearing the Space in your Mind

- *Find a quiet place and begin to breathe*

- Ask yourself: "What is distracting me from being present right now?"

- Give space to that distraction, whether it is an invasive thought, personal emotion, or someone else's emotion

- Say to yourself: "I am letting my distractions move through me as I ground myself in the present moment. Nothing is more important than right now."

- Breathe until you feel the distraction melt away into presence and mental clarity.

Re-Writing the Moment: A Short Meditation to Ease Emotional Pain of the Past

- Sit down with a journal and a pen and set your timer for 1 minute

- Take this 1 minute to write down any moment(s) of the past which have caused you a lot of pain

- After the minute is up, choose one of the painful moments, close your eyes, and begin to imagine the moment in a safe way. Be sure to keep breathing.

- When you open your eyes, take your pen and paper and re-imagine the painful moment. What do you wish had happened? How do you wish you could think about the moment now?

- After re-imagining the painful moment, remind yourself that this is a new moment. Everyone has painful memories, but you do not have to stay in spaces of the past, which are painful for you.

- Close your eyes, take a few more breaths, and say to yourself, "I release the pain of that moment of the past. This is a new moment, and I will move with it."

Re-claiming your Inner Power: A Short Meditation to Face Addiction

- Breathe into the moment, allowing yourself to think about the implications your addiction has on your life

- Without judgment, question your addiction. Ask yourself, "What has been left empty in me that I am trying to fill with this?" Listen for any emotions or past experiences of trauma, grief, or abandonment that arise. Allow them to be there.

- Say to yourself, "Now that I understand the root of my addiction, I can begin to be set free."

- With closed eyes, begin to breathe. With each breath, imagine your addiction's hold on you weakening and weakening until eventually, you have been released.

- Move forward into your life with the idea that your addiction's hold on you is loosening, day by day.

Letter to the Lost: A Short Meditation to Address Grief and Loss

- Sit down with a journal and a pen and take five deep breaths to bring you into the moment

- Allow someone you have lost to come to mind. This can be a relationship that has ended, someone who has died, etc.

- Close your eyes and breathe into the space this person has left empty within you. Allow yourself to experience any emotions that arise.

- When you open your eyes, take a few minutes to write what you wish you could have said to that person

- After you have finished your letter, close your eyes again. Tell your grief that it is okay for it to be there. With every breath, imagine yourself moving forward in your life, released from every regret you may have with someone you've lost

In with The Positive, Out with the Negative: A Short Breathing Technique

- Find a comfortable space and prepare to use the 5-5-7 breathing technique
- Breathe in for five counts and think of something positive you want to bring into this moment (kindness, peace, wisdom, etc.)
- Hold for five counts, allowing this positive thing to fill your body
- Exhale for seven counts, thinking of something negative you want to release from your body in this moment (stress, tension, selfishness, etc.)
- Begin again with a second emotion. Do this as many times as you like until you feel well-equipped with positive emotions and have released all negative ones

Space to Breathe: A Short Meditation to Gain Control over your Anxiety

- When you begin to feel anxious, step away, take a breath, and ground yourself in the moment by finding one thing you can see, one thing you can hear, and one thing you can feel. Focus deeply on each thing.

- Allow your anxiety space to exist. Remember, anxiety is the reaction your emotional brain has when it senses a threat. You can bring yourself back from catastrophe mode by using the rational brain to repeatedly remind yourself: "I am safe. I am in control. I am capable of being calm."

- Keep breathing and saying these rational-brained affirmations until you begin to feel your anxiety melt away

- Move into the next moment feeling calm, anxiety-free, and empowered

Emotion Coding: A Short Meditation to Bring you in Touch with your Emotions

- Find a quiet, comfortable place where you can easily connect with yourself

- Close your eyes and breathe deeply (you may use a breathing pattern if desired)

- Begin to travel inwards. Say to yourself, "I am ready to accept the emotions that are here."

- Wait patiently, focusing on the breath, and observing every emotion that rises to the surface.

- When an emotion arises, ask yourself a series of questions:

  1. "Is this emotion mine or someone else's?"
  2. "Does this emotion serve me or hold me back?"
  3. "What is this emotion trying to teach me?"
  4. "Should I release this emotion or put it into action?"

- When it comes to answering each question, listen to your intuition. The answers to each question are already within you. Do not question your natural answers.

- If you are being told to release an old or negative emotion, or an emotion that belongs to someone else, breathe and imagine it melting away with every exhale

- If you are being told to foster a positive emotion or a strong emotion that can create positive change in the world, sit with that, breathing, and being open to how that emotion can be useful.

The "I Love..." Gratitude Meditation (2-minute meditation)

- Find a private space, preferably one in front of a mirror
- Start a timer for 2 minutes
- For two minutes, speak out loud sentences of gratitude beginning with the words "I love..." ("I love my partner," "I love coffee," "I love my cat," "I love sunflowers," I love my mom," "I love to dance," "I love that I am healthy,").
- Say as many things as you can, one after the other. Do not think too much, simply let the things you love flow from your lips
- When the timer goes off, look in the mirror and say "And I love you," to yourself
- Feel the magic of gratitude transforming your life, your self-confidence, and your ability to be mindful

The Mindful Manifestation: A Short Meditation to Manifest what you Want in Life

- Sit down with a journal and pen

- Begin to cultivate mindfulness by bringing attention to your breath and any sensations in your body

- Ask yourself the question: "What do I want most in life?"

- As the answers start to come, open your eyes and begin to write your desires with the words "I manifest…" in front of them ("I manifest empathy." "I manifest peace of mind." "I manifest protection." "I manifest safety." "I manifest love." "I manifest awareness." "I manifest wisdom." "I manifest pure joy.")

- With each manifestation, close your eyes, and say it to yourself at least three times. Feel this manifestation become a part of your reality.

CPSIA information can be obtained
at www.ICGtesting.com
Printed in the USA
BVHW010430170221
600280BV00023B/44

9 781913 710828